Full Circle Fitness

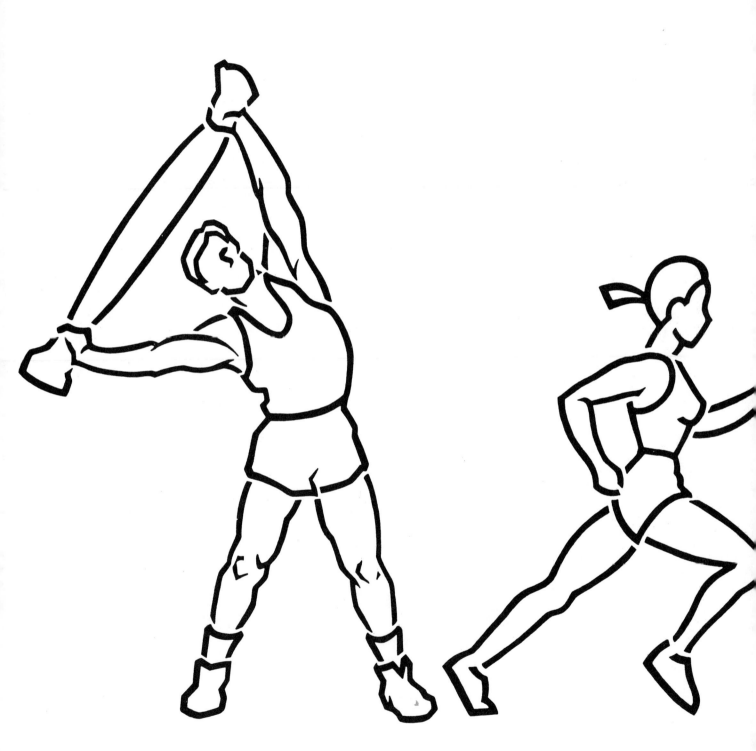

FULL CIRCLE FITNESS
Be Your Own Personal Trainer

REBECCA EASTMAN
with Patricia Ryan

Photographs by Tony Costa
Illustrations by Lianne Auck

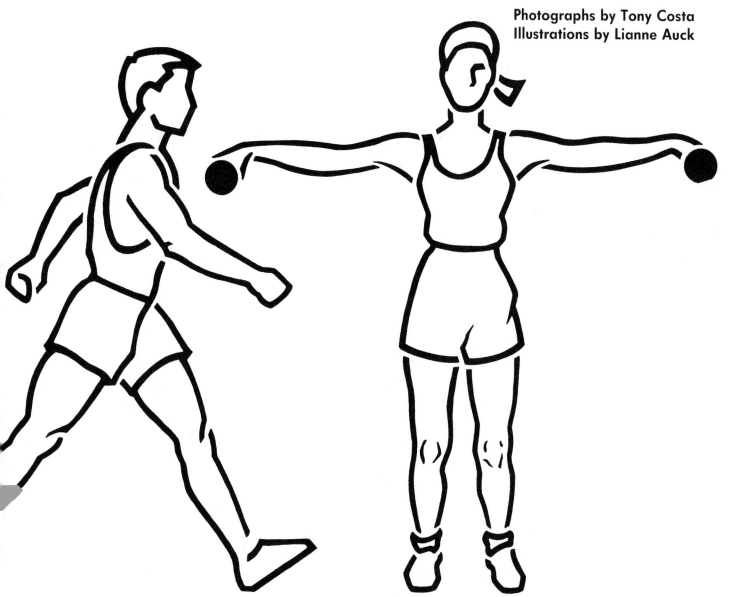

William Morrow and Company, Inc., New York

Dedication

There is a body of knowledge that indicates diet and exercise can modify the risks associated with disease. The management of illness lies in preventive health practices as well as medical treatment.

This book is dedicated to my father whose generation was not aware of the impact mindful nutrition and regular exercise can have on the quality of life. His experience inspired me to write this book.

A Note of Caution

Before beginning this, or any other, exercise program, it is advisable to obtain the approval and recommendations of your physician. While you are on this, or any, exercise program, it is advisable to visit your physician for periodic monitoring. This program is intended for adults in good health.

The author and publisher of this book disclaim any liability or loss in connection with the exercises and advice herein.

Copyright © 1990 by Rebecca Eastman Full Circle Fitness®

Library of Congress Cataloging-in-Publication Data

Eastman, Rebecca.
Full circle fitness.
1. Exercise. 2. Physical fitness. I. Ryan, Patricia.
II. Title.
RA781.E22 1989   613.7   88-34479
ISBN 0-688-07419-7

Printed in the United States of America

First Edition

1 2 3 4 5 6 7 8 9 10

BOOK DESIGN BY GARRY TOSTI

Acknowledgments

When I put Full Circle Fitness Training into book format, my primary concern was time management. The individual contributions from the following people were invaluable. They deserve my sincere thanks for their support of this book.

First, to my mentor, Anne-Marie Bennstrom, for the guidance and knowledge she has shared over the years, my unbroken respect and love.

To Patricia Ryan, editor at *IDEA: The Association of Fitness Professionals*, for her help with organizing and rewriting the material. From the outline inception to the final draft, her creative energy, talent, and commitment brought my personal training programs to a concrete text.

To Dick Cotton, exercise physiologist at Scripps Clinic and Research Foundation, for providing clarity, detail, and integrity to the final manuscript.

To my editor, Jennifer Williams, whose enthusiasm kept me focused, productive, and afloat throughout the project.

To Robbie Capp, my copy editor and guardian angel of the final manuscript, and to Garry Tosti, my book designer, who saved this project with his extraordinary talent and patience; a standing ovation for a job well done.

To illustrator Lianne Auck and photographer Tony Costa for their outstanding visualization of the exercises and the personal training experience.

My sincere thanks to those who shared their hearts: Leslie Belzberg, Carole Ellis, Bruce Gilbert, Emese and Leonard Green, Bette Light, Stacie Hunt, Karen Montgomery, Harriett Selwyn, Alfre and Roderick Spencer, Lily Tomlin, and George Watson.

To those who encouraged me: Bill Adler, Karen Kearns, Sylvia Merschel, Donald Perry, Barbara Rowes, and Eva Shaw.

And to those who gave time and energy as co-workers of Full Circle Fitness: Lynn Forbes, Glen Gaither, Christopher Hall, Kim Kaminski, Russell Kohn, Wayne Lowder, Bob Miko, Don Parris, Monika Roth, and Liz Sibert.

Finally I give special thanks to Betty Eastman, my mother, who not only typed chapters and charts into the wee hours of the morning, but also shared her insights to bring this to final form.

CONTENTS

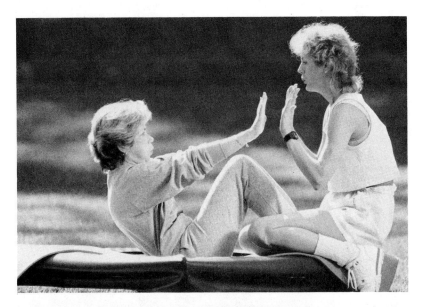

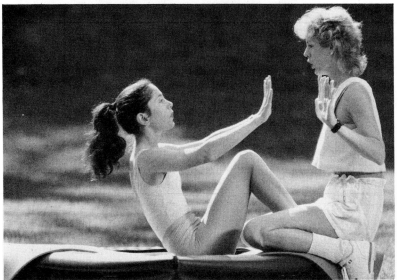

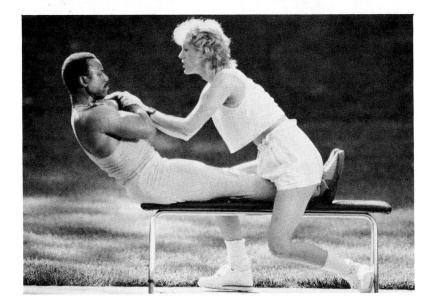

1

WHAT IS PERSONAL FITNESS TRAINING?

I am a personal fitness trainer. I work on a one-to-one basis with women and men from all backgrounds. I have worked with corporate executives and small-business owners, secretaries and full-time mothers, actresses and producers. All my new clients, whether they're completely sedentary or exercise regulars, want the same thing: to look good and feel great.

Why do they choose me for a trainer? There are no mysterious fitness "tricks" inside my gym bag. But there is a lot of knowledge about fitness and motivation that I've learned through both formal education and years of experience. I work one-to-one with each client, developing a personalized program and teaching exercise skills that eventually allow them to continue the program without me. Once they learn the skills, the energy, vitality, and self-esteem that comes from being fit enhances their lives long after they're on their own.

While you follow the program described in this book, we'll work together so that you, too, can maintain a lifetime of fitness. I've named the lifetime fitness programs "A Handle on Health" and "The Competitive Edge." To achieve these exercise lifestyles, I'll safely prepare and gradually progress you with an exercise program tailored for your

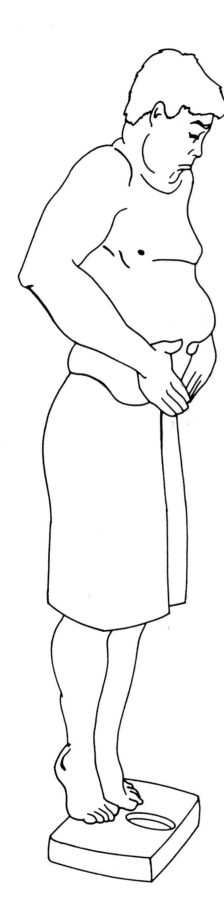

current level of fitness. Plus, as with all my clients, you'll learn to set goals, not expectations, as you refine the skills that enable you to make fitness a regular part of your life.

One of my clients, a fifty-six-year-old clothing manufacturer named Jack, recently remarked that he never thought he'd be exercising at all—and certainly didn't expect to be successful at it. It wasn't even Jack's idea to begin a fitness program. He'd received one month of personal training as a gift from his family, who felt he had everything—except control of his health. That start gave Jack enough motivation to continue. After six months of following the program, Jack lost twenty-five pounds.

But best of all, Jack realized that exercise was no longer an unpleasant chore that had to be endured in order to avoid reprimands from his doctor and his wife. He *looked forward* to exercise once it became part of his lifestyle. Jack's consistent fitness habits helped him lose weight and feel younger. No overnight miracle diet or gimmick can deliver those results.

You can have the same experience Jack did. Once you start exercising with a **Full Circle Fitness** program designed for whole-body exercise, you'll be stronger and firmer, lose unnecessary pounds and inches, gain aerobic endurance, and be more flexible. You'll also experience increased alertness and vitality, with plenty of energy to enjoy leisure activities and contend with life's challenges.

Finding a Fitness Lifestyle

Before a person formally enrolls in my program, we have a long chat to review his or her personal history and possible expectations. We need to discuss a few issues because, for a personalized training program to be effective, it's necessary to work together. Before you begin the program, it's a good idea to investigate your own motives. This will allow you to set goals and examine weaknesses or patterns of behavior.

These questions are usually raised at the first meeting:

Why do you want to start exercising? *Maybe it's to lose ten or fifteen pounds. The lure of winning a race or improving your figure for a new love interest can make you serious about getting in shape. Perhaps you've started exercising, but aren't sure if it's safe or how to stick with it. It could be that you are feeling sluggish, or that a doctor has prescribed regular exercise. Your goals and present physical condition help determine the training program to get you started.*

What do you expect to be the result of exercise? *Many people want to lose twenty pounds in a month; others want spectacular increases in muscle size in a few weeks. Unfortunately, neither of these expectations is realistic in this amount of time. In reality, you will see measurable improvements in health and physique slowly and steadily, over months. Set goals, not expectations!*

When are you going to fit exercise into an already hectic schedule? *Keeping an appointment to exercise three days a week can be a real stickler for many of my clients. One reason people hire me is because our meetings become scheduled events. We set aside time for a one-hour meeting, rain or shine, every week. Scheduling time for your program will get you real results.*

Will you stay with the commitment you make for at least three months, even if you don't see remarkable changes immediately? *Since there are no instant results, it can be hard work sticking with it. Not every workout, particularly those at the beginning, will be a joyful adventure in athleticism. Consistent effort will be rewarded in four to eight weeks.*

Once you answer these questions, you'll have an idea of what your exercise goals are and how you will try to achieve them. These realizations can reinforce your determination to experience the rewards of exercise.

When I told Lynn, who has a high-stress, sit-down job, that she could lose six to eight pounds—not twenty—in a month, she was disappointed and felt a little let down. After all, I was a personal trainer and I could work miracles. But after we talked about the "whys," Lynn decided to try a regular exercise program since strict dieting and spa-hopping hadn't kept the weight off.

Lynn started exercising, lost extra pounds and inches, maintained her weight loss, and stuck with her exercise plan once she was on her own. She discovered she was getting a lot more than just a thinner body. The commitment necessary to achieve her goal was just as important and fulfilling, and exercise was fun! A year later, Lynn's not thinking about what the scale reads every morning. She is taking fitness vacations, participating in sports with friends, and exercising regularly by walking briskly before work or catching a lunchtime aerobics class. She is much more relaxed and satisfied with herself than she was when she had her first consultation with me. Quite an accomplishment for a person who was desk-bound, stressed, and overweight.

Lynn's determination to lose weight started her on the

training program, but it was her discovery of the health benefits and the fun of regular exercise that kept her active after her initial goal had been accomplished. The exercise lifestyle that Lynn has achieved is the same one you will be working toward. The charts at right represent a year of **Full Circle Fitness.**

The **Gain, Train,** and **Maintain** programs in this book are designed to prepare you for a future of exercise with A Handle on Health or The Competitive Edge. Each one is planned for a specific level of physical fitness designed to achieve your immediate goals. Depending on your current level of fitness and your consistency in making time for exercise, it will take approximately four to six months to generate a lifestyle exercise program. That's all.

A Handle on Health is preventive health care with a routine that will help you modify your risk of heart disease with only four hours of exercise a week and give you a sense of well-being that can be felt every day. It provides more than a body weight that's comfortable and muscles that are strong and flexible enough to keep everyday chores easy. Healthy people radiate a youthful appearance and a cheerful, relaxed attitude.

The Competitive Edge encompasses all these health benefits, plus it allows you to focus on sports conditioning. This program intensifies strength training and adds two 45-minute endurance sessions per week. These qualities will serve you well in the boardroom as well as on the sports field.

A great advantage to having both these programs is that you can switch between them depending on your goals and interests. If you are already very fit, you can begin A Handle on Health or The Competitive Edge today.

For example, Lynn began at the **Gain** level because she had not exercised in the last few years and was twenty pounds overweight. It took her three hours a week for six weeks to complete *The **Gain** Program.* She then graduated to *The Train Program,* where she also exercised for three hours a week for six weeks, but at a different level and with some new exercises. Then Lynn progressed to *The Maintain Program* for twelve weeks where she added one 30-minute endurance session to her three-hours-a-week schedule. In just six months of regular training, once sedentary and overweight Lynn had gained the knowledge and conditioning level to reach A Handle on Health. In this lifestyle exercise program, she now schedules four hours a week for exercise.

Where Do I Begin?

Once you have answered the critical question, "Where do I begin?" the charts below progress your program to improve your capacity. Depending on your current level of fitness it will take approximately four to six months to generate a lifestyle exercise program. The Train and Maintain programs have different exercise guidelines so be sure to follow the chart that is recommended in your beginning exercise program. If you are already exercising three times per week for six months you can begin with A Handle on Health or The Competitive Edge today. If however, you wish to plateau your activity at any of the programs you will still realize many of the health benefits of physical activity.

The Competitive Edge—lifestyle exercise
Total weekly training time = 4½ hours
Extra weight training and aerobics allow the dedicated exerciser to enhance strength and endurance along with motor and concentration skills.

A Handle on Health—lifestyle exercise
Total weekly training time = 4 hours
A robust balance of aerobic endurance, muscle strength and shape, flexibility and relaxation make this stage a life-long habit and a wise investment in preventive health care.

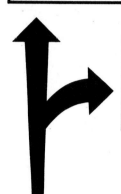

Maintain—12–16 Weeks
Total weekly training time = 3½ hours
Muscle size and strength become defined, weight loss goals are coming closer, and stamina levels allow you to add aerobic sessions. You can diversify into a variety of aerobic activities or increase the time in strength and flexibility training.

Train—6–10 Weeks
Total weekly training time = 3 hours
You can improve considerably here, and be able to add additional aerobic exercise because of increased stamina. How fast you increase the duration and intensity depends on your age. For each decade over age 30, it takes about one week longer for your body to adapt.

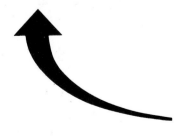

Gain—6 Weeks
Total weekly training time = 3 hours
The length of time for initial conditioning depends a great deal on your current fitness level, your exercise history, and how well your body responds to the exercise training. When starting out, it is best to be very conservative to give your body plenty of time to adjust and to avoid excess muscle soreness, injury, and frustration. By the end of this time period, you'll start to lose pounds and inches, increase muscle tone, strength and flexibility, and improve stamina.

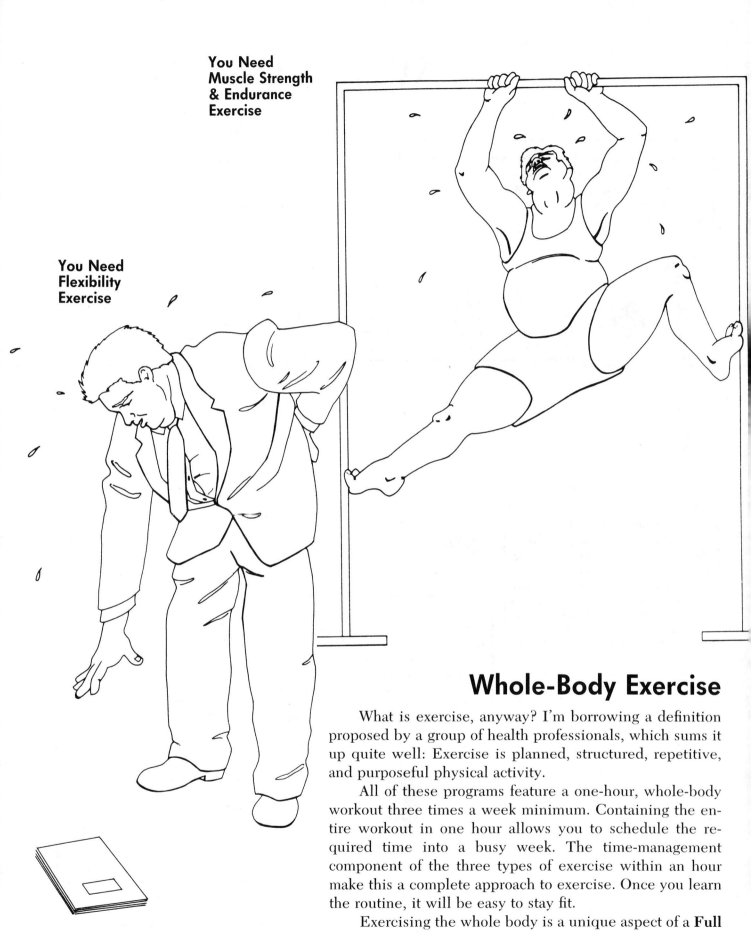

**You Need
Muscle Strength
& Endurance
Exercise**

**You Need
Flexibility
Exercise**

Whole-Body Exercise

What is exercise, anyway? I'm borrowing a definition proposed by a group of health professionals, which sums it up quite well: Exercise is planned, structured, repetitive, and purposeful physical activity.

All of these programs feature a one-hour, whole-body workout three times a week minimum. Containing the entire workout in one hour allows you to schedule the required time into a busy week. The time-management component of the three types of exercise within an hour make this a complete approach to exercise. Once you learn the routine, it will be easy to stay fit.

Exercising the whole body is a unique aspect of a **Full**

Circle Fitness session. Some exercises concentrate on only one part of your body. For example, running trains the muscles of your legs, heart, and lungs but it ignores the arms and chest. To insure whole-body training, the following improvements will be made with three types of exercise:

Aerobic Exercise The primary component for most programs is the aerobic exercise. Aerobic exercise utilizes oxygen and stimulates the supply of oxygen to the heart and the exercised muscles. Any activity that utilizes major muscle groups continuously at an intensity high enough to stimulate a change in the body, but not so high that it can't be sustained for at least 20 minutes, is aerobic exercise. Popular aerobic activities are walking, cycling, aerobic dancing, jogging, rowing, swimming, and cross-country skiing. Unlike daily interest payments at the bank, aerobic endurance can't be compounded. What you gain in six weeks, you can lose in three, if you stop exercising.

Aerobic exercise is the key to overall good health. It provides the energy and stress release that enhances daily living. It controls weight and body-fat levels, fights the risk factors of coronary heart disease, and generally keeps your metabolic motor well-tuned.

Flexibility Exercise Flexibility is determined by the elasticity of the muscles, and the tendons and ligaments that attach them to the bones. It is defined by the range of motion a body part has as it moves around a joint.

The ability to move limbs through their full range of motion counteracts stress on the body, which makes work and play easier and helps keep you injury-free. Flexibility allows you to move with coordination and ease.

Muscle Strength and Endurance Exercise Muscle strength is measured by the amount of force you can apply against resistance as when you lift a heavy box. Muscle endurance is the ability to use your strength over a period of time, as when raking leaves. To acquire muscle strength and muscle endurance, you must move your muscles through their range of motion against resistance such as your own body weight, or the resistance provided by free weights or machines.

Muscle strength and muscle endurance work together to make it easier to climb stairs, carry objects, and perform any task or sport that requires sustained exertion. Toned, firm muscles also give your body physical beauty and muscle definition.

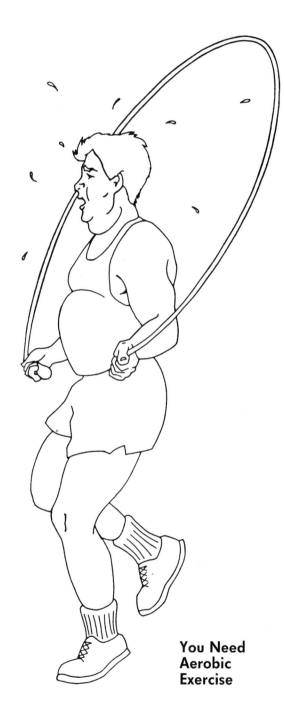

You Need Aerobic Exercise

The Time-Management Component

These types of exercise will be combined into your one-hour routine as shown on the clock. Every one-hour exercise session runs clockwise with warm-up flexibility stretches, aerobic exercise, muscle strength exercise, and cool-down flexibility stretches.

Flexibility stretches will start the exercise hour. The aerobic session follows flexibility and begins with three minutes of low-intensity activity to prepare you for aerobic conditioning. The aerobic session ends with another three minutes of gradually decreasing intensity to safely decrease your heart rate. Strength exercises follow the aerobic conditioning period to work major muscle groups. Flexibility exercises, known as cool-down stretches, complete a safe and effective whole-body workout. Just follow the clock in your program for a comprehensive approach to physical fitness.

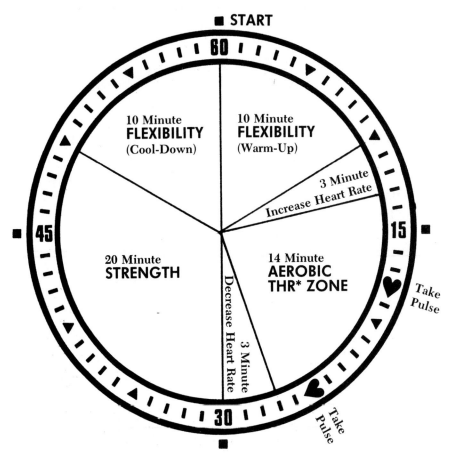

A Sample Exercise Hour

*Training Heart Rate

You Can Do It!

When faced with the reality of making a commitment to regular exercise each week and understanding enough about exercise theory to plan an effective program, even the most motivated person may falter. Exercise seems simplistic, but it takes effort and knowledge to do it right so that you can ultimately achieve your goals and have fun while doing it.

What's the alternative? For many people it seems to be a steady downward spiral into overweight, muscle weakness, possible heart disease, chronic fatigue, and all the other physical losses that we call "just getting older." But it doesn't have to be that way.

Medical authorities are discovering that these so-called signs of aging are instead signs of inactivity. For example, a study of the relationship between health and exercise examined 4,500 men aged forty-five years and older. The active sixty-five-year-old men had approximately the same physical capabilities as the sedentary forty-five-year-olds. The sixty-five-year-old men had reduced their "biological age" by twenty years by just staying active! There's no reason why you have to sit around and watch your body deteriorate while you watch television. You can do something about it.

I train a couple in their late forties who originally called me because they wanted to prepare for a hiking trek in the Himalayas. They were smart enough not to go without some physical conditioning. We met every other day at 6:30 A.M. for an hour of whole-body exercise that included stationary cycling, rowing and jogging, light weight lifting, and stretching. That 6:30 A.M. workout required a lot of effort on their part. They own two major corporations and spend very full days—sedentary, but full—attending board meetings, organizing and directing, and aiding charity events. Jogging on cold, foggy mornings is not easy. But they had a *goal*, a purpose that made them keep their exercise commitment.

You can imagine how excited I was when I answered the phone one night and amid the crackling, buzzing noise, realized they were calling from Kathmandu, Nepal, to thank me and share news of their success with the trek. They enjoyed themselves tremendously because they had the foresight to prepare physically and mentally. Exercise became a specific goal and the realization of that goal became a part of their lives. Today they are still training and planning a spring trek in the Andes mountains.

People make appointments with me to keep appointments with themselves. You must do the same and be willing to schedule a regular exercise time into your life. I can prescribe a wide range of programs, but the keys are within you. You have to desire a change, you have to be determined. Basically, you have to hang in there for the first six weeks until you start to see real results, which will be motivating in themselves. But, you have to make health and fitness as important a priority as your job and your family. Our bodies age as a result of disuse, degenerative disease, and the natural aging process. Two of these three can be reduced or completely reversed with a program of regular physical activity.

You can do it!

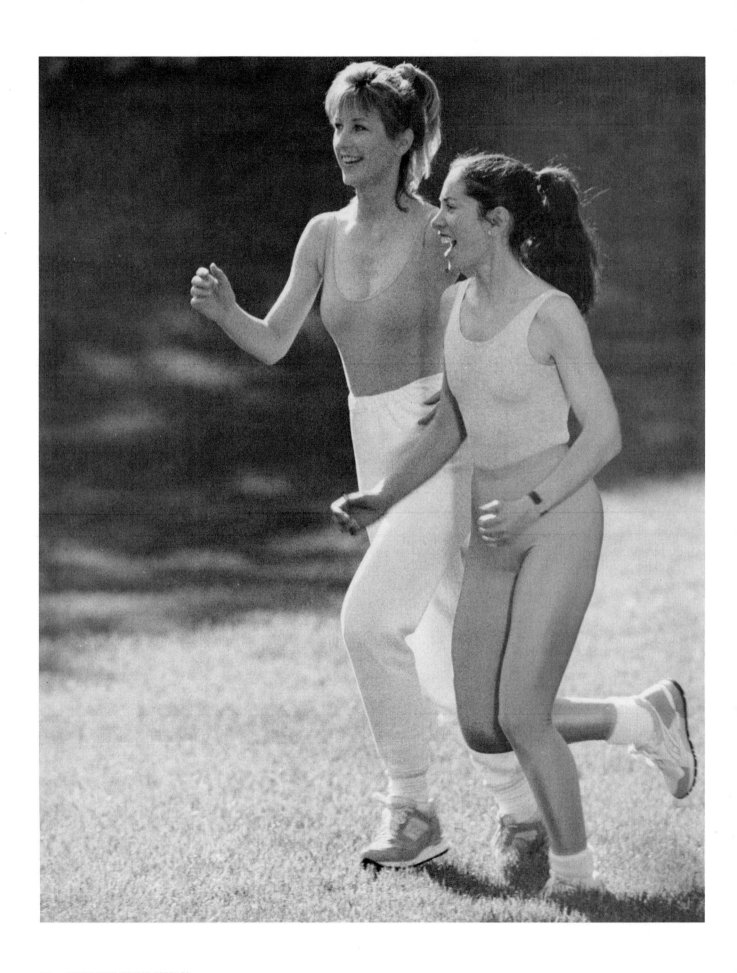

2

WHAT'S YOUR FITNESS PROFILE?

During the first appointment with a new client, we cover a lot of ground. First we discuss goals and how the programs are designed. (Personally, I think everyone's a little relieved not to be sweating bullets in the first ten minutes.)

After answering any questions, we begin to evaluate the client's current health status and level of fitness. Here the person has to do some work. First, that means filling out a health-history questionnaire.

The health-history questionnaire that follows will help you determine if you should see a doctor before beginning your exercise program. If you discover a risk for coronary heart disease, or are doubtful about your state of health, it's a good idea to have a physical examination.

When a person has exercise limitations, I follow the physician's guidelines when establishing the program. Perhaps the individual must start very slowly, exercising at a very low intensity, and for short periods of time. As the person improves, the program will modify as the doctor monitors progress. This person's program, too, will contain flexibility, aerobic, and strength training.

Determining Your Health History

General Health and Lifestyle

1. Describe your present health status:
   Very Good___ Average___ Poor___ Very Poor___

2. How would you describe your energy level?
   High___ Average___ Low___

3. Do you consider yourself:
   Underweight___ Normal Weight___ Overweight___
   Very Overweight ___

4. What was/is your weight:
   5 years ago_____ 1 year ago_____ Today_____

5. Do you diet three or more times per year?
   Yes___ No___

6. Do you smoke? Yes___ No___ If so, for how many years?_____
   How much?_____ (packs/pipes/cigars) per day

7. Did you formerly smoke? Yes___ No___
   When did you quit?_____

8. Are you presently engaging in any type of exercise
   or recreational activity? Yes___ No___
   Type of exercise_____
   How long (minutes)_____
   How often (days per week)_____
   How hard (heart rate)_____
   For how long (months/years)_____

9. In what type of physical activity have you participated
   in the past?_____
   How long (minutes)_____
   How often (days per week)_____
   How hard (heart rate)_____
   When did you quit? (months/years)_____

10. Do you exercise more than six days per week? Yes___ No___

11. Do you consider your day:
    Sedentary___ Moderately Active___ Very Active___

12. How many hours do you spend sitting each day?_____

13. Do you consider your day stressful?
    Yes___ No___ Sometimes ___

14. Do you handle stress/anxiety with:
    ___ Alcohol   ___ Exercise   ___ Cigarettes
    ___ Tranquilizers   ___ Television   ___ Sweets
    ___ Drugs   ___ Coffee   ___ Food

Cardiopulmonary Assessment

15. Have you ever had any of the following? (If yes, consult your
    physician before beginning an exercise program)

Yes	No	Don't Know	
○	○	○	Heart Attack
○	○	○	High Blood Pressure
○	○	○	Abnormal EKG
○	○	○	Skipped or Rapid Heartbeat
○	○	○	High Cholesterol
○	○	○	Rheumatic Fever
○	○	○	Diabetes

16. Have you ever experienced chest discomfort? Yes___ No___

Musculoskeletal Assessment

17. Have you ever had any of the following? (If yes, consult your
    physician before beginning an exercise program)

Yes	No	Don't Know	
○	○	○	Arthritis
○	○	○	Osteoporosis
○	○	○	Joint Discomfort or Injury: (shoulder, elbow, hip, knee, ankle, foot, etc.)

Back Pain

18. Do you have back pain? Yes___ No___ (If yes, consult your
    physician before beginning an exercise program)
    If yes, how often? Every day___ With exercise___
    Does this limit your ability to exercise? Yes___ No___

Family History

19. Please list all family members who have/had a history of
    heart disease, strokes, high blood pressure, or diabetes:

Relationship	Type of Disease	Age at Diagnosis	Age at Death
_____	_____	_____	_____
_____	_____	_____	_____
_____	_____	_____	_____
_____	_____	_____	_____

(If any members are younger than fifty, consult your physician
before beginning an exercise program.)

Risk Factors You Can and Can't Modify

Exercise along with prudent nutrition does a lot of valuable things while improving your appearance and controlling your weight. For example, studies have shown that low-impact exercise such as walking, cross-country skiing, and dance exercise, is a front-line defense against calcium loss in the bones, which leads to osteoporosis. Activity such as stretching and water exercise can counteract the crippling effects of arthritis.

When a client and I review a health history, I generally explain the factors that can lead to poor health, and how exercise can affect them.

Exercise can significantly modify the risk factors for the leading cause of death in the United States: *coronary heart disease*, known as CHD, which incapacitates or kills over 600,000 people each year. The physical problems, or risk factors, that precede CHD are serious in themselves. You *can modify* one set of risk factors. They are:

Inactivity	Cigarette Smoking
Obesity	Diabetes
High Blood Pressure	Stress
High Cholesterol	

The good news is that not only can you reduce these risk factors, but you have a much stronger defense against the ones you can't modify: age, gender, and family history.

Inactivity A recent review of the risk factor literature by the Centers for Disease Control revealed that *inactivity* leads the list of risk factors. Not being active is hard on your heart, body, and mental outlook. It increases your percentage of body fat and weakens the efficiency of your muscles, joints, and circulatory system. Plus it speeds the aging process. A sedentary lifestyle makes you vulnerable to disease, injury, and fatigue; it decreases your ability to concentrate, and it can lower your self-esteem. But don't get too depressed. A program of regular exercise can have a tremendously positive impact on these conditions. Besides, when you "use it" you won't "lose it" as you get older.

Obesity Even though dieting is a national obsession, excessive body fat is still a major health concern for many people. When you eat more calories than your body needs for energy, the excess is stored as fat. Regular exercise, combined with a sensible diet, is the most successful means of

Coronary Risk Factors

The major coronary risk factors are:

1. History of high blood pressure.
2. Elevated total cholesterol/HDL (high-density lipoprotein) cholesterol ratio.
3. Cigarette smoking.
4. Abnormal resting EKG (electrocardiogram)—including evidence of an old heart attack, enlarged heart, lack of oxygen to the heart muscle, or irregularities in the heart's rhythm.
5. Family history of coronary or other artery disease prior to age fifty.
6. Diabetes.

According to the American College of Sports Medicine, you should visit the doctor if you match one of the following descriptions:

Apparently healthy individuals, without the above risk factors at age forty-five or older should have an exercise EKG to establish an effective and safe exercise program.

If you are older than thirty-five and have one or more of the above risk factors, your physician may require an exercise EKG.

Persons at any age with symptoms that suggest coronary, pulmonary, or metabolic disease should have a physician-supervised exercise EKG prior to beginning a vigorous exercise program.

You might want to obtain a copy of the health tests the doctor performs so that you can keep a record of this information.

Weight Range Formula

Until you have your percent of body fat measured, you can estimate healthy body weight using the following formula.

Women start with 100 pounds for 5 feet of height, then add 5 pounds for every inch of height over 5 feet; 15 pounds *above and below* this number will give you a 30-pound weight range.

Men start with 106 pounds for 5 feet of height and add 6 pounds for every inch of height over 5 feet; 15 pounds *above and below* this number will give you a 30-pound weight range.

The lower 10 pounds of this range are an estimation for a small frame, the middle ten pounds are an estimation for a medium frame, and the upper 10 pounds are an estimation for a large-frame person.

Examples:

- *Woman* 5'5" = 100 + 25 = 125 lbs. Weight range 110–140 lbs.: small frame, 110–120 lbs.; medium frame, 120–130 lbs.; large frame, 130–140 lbs.
- *Man* 5'10" = 106 + 60 = 166 lbs. Weight range 151–181 lbs.: small frame, 151–161 lbs.; medium frame, 161–171 lbs.; large frame, 171–181 lbs.

Don't forget that these numbers are an estimation of a *range of weight* for your height and frame.

Borderline reading: 140/90—see your doctor to control your blood pressure.
Ideal reading: 130/80 or less—your blood pressure is normal.

---

achieving and, most importantly, *maintaining desirable body weight*. Aerobic exercise encourages the body to burn fat for fuel. Exercise also makes changes in the muscles that enhance your ability to burn fat.

"Body composition" is the term that describes the ratio of body fat to lean muscle, bones, and organs. Most experts recommend that adult women maintain between 18–27 percent of the body weight as fat weight. Women over 30 percent fat are considered obese. Adult men should have a body-fat percentage between 13–20 percent. For men, over 25 percent fat is considered obese. It can be equally unhealthy to fall below 12 percent fat for women, and 7 percent for men. A person who has too little body fat risks a loss of energy, menstrual cycle, and bone mass, increasing the risk for osteoporosis.

The most accurate method of determining your body fat percentage is underwater weighing, but a fairly accurate and easier method is measuring skinfolds at various places on the body using calipers. Both require a qualified specialist. A sports medicine center or hospital can refer you to centers for body-fat measurement.

Fat plus muscle, bones, and organs equals your total body weight. So-called "ideal" weight depends on your bone structure and amount of musculature as well as your height and sex. Regardless of how you determine your ideal body weight, it is unrealistic to try to force yourself to maintain a specific body weight. I've found that most people range from three to five pounds above or below an ideal weight. That's well within reason and I suggest you allow yourself the same leeway.

High Blood Pressure/Hypertension Blood pressure varies from minute to minute, going up with activity or excitement and going down at rest. High blood pressure increases the work load on your heart and is hard on the blood vessels. Sometimes referred to as "the silent killer," the symptoms usually occur only after irreversible damage has been done, and with no warning signs. This is why frequent check-ups are important and why medication may be prescribed to control your blood pressure. Ideally, high blood pressure should be controlled with diet, smoking cessation, weight loss, and exercise. Researchers have discovered that active people have lower heart rates and resting blood pressures than sedentary people, which means their hearts don't have to work as hard.

High Cholesterol A fatty substance manufactured by the body, cholesterol is necessary for normal body function. Most excess cholesterol is carried away with the blood flow, but some is deposited on the walls of the arteries. This excess narrows the channels, blocking the flow of blood to the heart, brain, or limbs.

The types of cholesterol are HDL or "good cholesterol" and LDL or "bad cholesterol." HDL helps protect you from the buildup of the more harmful LDL cholesterol, therefore higher levels (greater than 25 percent of total cholesterol) are considered desirable.

Your doctor can tell you where you can have your blood tested for cholesterol levels, or you can take advantage of testing centers that offer this service. Losing excess weight and increasing physical activity help lower cholesterol levels. So does decreasing your intake of dietary cholesterol (it's in foods from animal sources) and minimizing your intake of saturated fats in red meats, and palm and coconut oils. Additional soluble dietary fiber—such as oat bran, bananas, apples, green beans, and legumes—is also helpful.

Cigarette Smoking Are you dying for a cigarette? You literally may be doing just that. Smoking elevates blood pressure, impedes circulation by constricting arteries, increases adrenaline, and damages the walls of the arteries. It's horrifying to realize that carbon dioxide takes the place of oxygen in your red blood cells when you inhale cigarette smoke. If you smoke, you are increasing your chance of a heart attack. The more you smoke, the greater the risk. No, those low-tar, low-nicotine cigarettes don't lower your chance of heart disease.

But exercise can help you kick the habit. A study of the participants at Atlanta's Peachtree Road Race showed that 76 percent of the women and 81 percent of the men who were smokers when they started running quit as a result of their new activity.

Diabetes Diabetes can result from either your lifestyle or your heredity. Diabetes falls into two groups: Type I is usually hereditary and requires insulin; the much more common Type II is typically acquired by someone who is over forty and overweight. Frequently, Type II diabetes can be prevented with low-intensity exercise, prudent nutrition, and weight control.

If you are at risk or currently have this disease, consult your doctor before beginning any exercise program. Your

---

Total cholesterol is made up of LDL, HDL, and two other insignificant types. These levels pertain to men and women:
- Ideal total cholesterol is 200 (mg %) or less.
- Moderately high cholesterol is 200–240 (mg %).
- High cholesterol is anything greater than 240 (mg %).

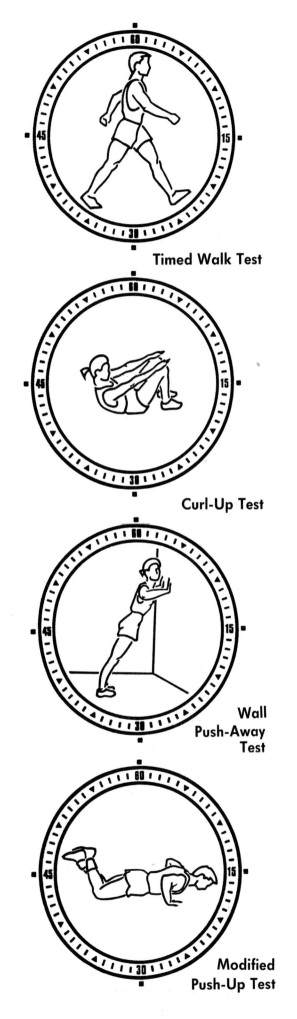

Timed Walk Test

Curl-Up Test

Wall
Push-Away
Test

Modified
Push-Up Test

doctor will probably suggest using a glucometer to measure blood glucose levels before and after exercise. Partner exercising is recommended.

Stress While a certain amount of stress is necessary to make the body function and stimulate us into action, too much emotional stress can make us tense and unhappy. Although we live in the twentieth century, humans still react with caveman primitiveness to the hundreds of irritations that occur every day. Besides unhappiness, these responses include muscle tension, elevated heart and blood-pressure rates, and increased cholesterol levels.

Physical activity and relaxation are the tools that help manage the stress we accumulate. Exercise relaxes muscles and lowers heart-rate and cholesterol levels. Plus, aerobic exercise encourages the release of endorphins, the body's natural pain killers and mood elevators.

Age and Gender These factors are important in determining your exercise program and the intensity at which you should exercise. As age increases, you increase the risk of heart disease. Scientific studies have shown that men are at greater risk of heart attacks than women, particularly premenopausal women.

Family History If family members (parents, aunts, uncles, brothers, sisters, and grandparents) have had heart disease or a stroke at an age earlier than fifty years, then your risk for heart disease increases.

Your Fitness Assessment

We can measure your physical fitness with the timed walk or step test, flexibility, and muscle endurance tests. There are good reasons for taking these simple exercise tests that determine your current level of fitness. These assessments help you choose an exercise program that is best

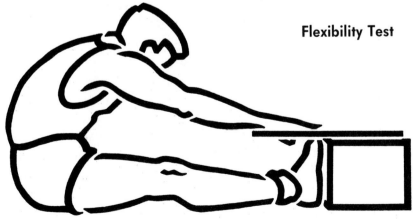

Flexibility Test

suited to your individual level. By knowing how fit you are today, you will be able to measure your progress and compare your performance at a later date. Watching your progress can be an important motivational tool.

All of the clients I train start with these fitness assessments. You'll find them in the Appendix. I strongly advise that you use these non-strenuous tests to measure your physical fitness because they are so valuable in the long run.

Once you have completed the fitness assessments, record the results on the personal fitness progress chart that is also included in the Appendix. This will allow you to easily keep an ongoing record of your progress as you repeat the tests periodically through your programs.

The last step in assessing your fitness is weighing in and taking your measurements with a tape measure. Light or no clothing and bare feet are recommended. To be accurate, measure at the same place each time. A tape measure is much better than a scale for keeping track of weight loss and increases in muscle size because it more accurately measures loss of body fat. Record your measurements and weight on the chart you'll find in the Appendix.

The Step Test

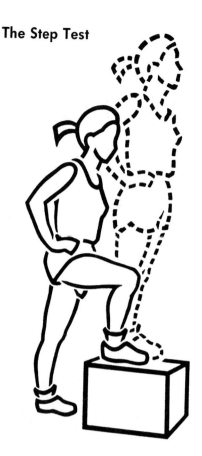

The Fitness Profile

The Gain Program For the person who hasn't been active in the last six months or has never been active or desires 15 to 30 pounds of weight loss or scored low in the Fitness Assessment.

The Train Program For the person who exercises once in a while or desires 5 to 15 pounds of weight loss or scored low to mid-range in the Fitness Assessment.

The Maintain Program For the person who exercises two times per week or exercises regularly on the weekends or scored mid to upper range in the Fitness Assessment or already has an ideal weight range.

A Handle on Health For the person who exercises three or more times per week for a period of six months or desires to maintain a state of optimal health or scored in the upper range on the Fitness Assessment.

The Competitive Edge For the person who exercises three or more times per week for a period of six months or wants to maintain health and enhance sport skills or scored in the upper range on the Fitness Assessment.

Your Fitness Profile

When you combine the information from your health history, fitness assessments, and measurements, you have objective data about your current state of physical conditioning. These facts, together with your present exercise habits, will indicate where you should begin exercising. To simplify the decision, match your results with the characteristics outlined on *The Fitness Profile*. Pay special attention to your current level of activity because it is a critical factor.

The Fitness Profile is a tool we'll be using regularly. Exercise is progressive, and you won't stay at the same level of conditioning forever. Not only does it tell you where to start, but when you take the fitness assessments periodically, the profile can guide you as you progress to the next program. Exercising at the proper level encourages success, and *The Fitness Profile* tailors the programs specifically for you.

If you are undecided between two programs, pick the lower of the choices. After participating for six sessions, if the program feels too easy then progress to the next level of that program.

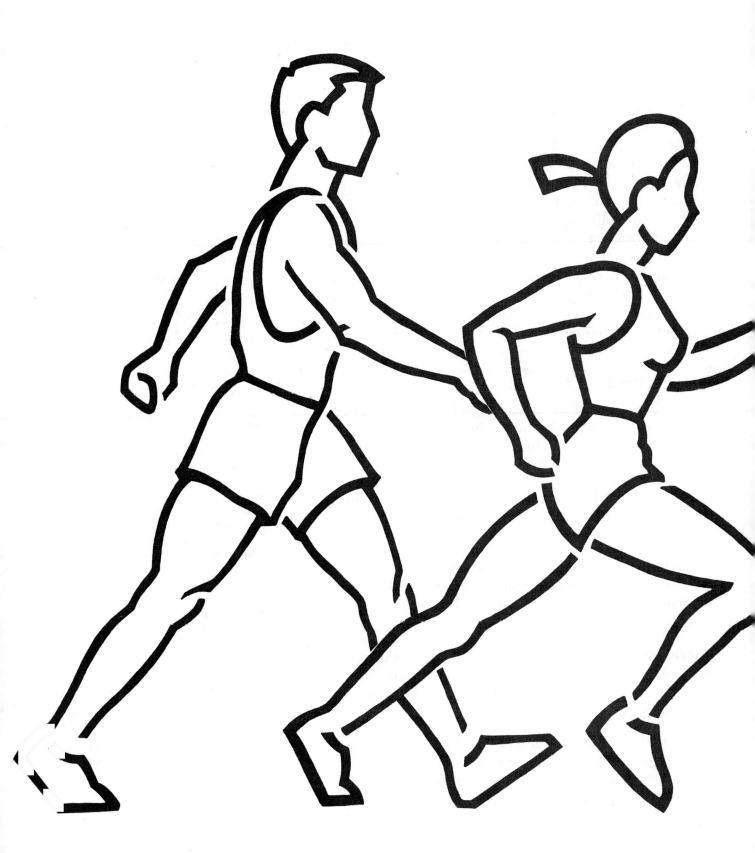

YOUR EXERCISE PRESCRIPTION

3

An exercise prescription is a plan that helps you become fit—it has nothing to do with medication. It's called a "prescription" because you have to follow certain principles for the exercise program to work, just like following a doctor's prescription will improve your health. The scientific principles that underlie any sound exercise plan have been determined through the research of exercise physiologists, physicians, epidemiologists, and others. Of course, the observations of sports coaches—the original personal trainers—have helped point the way, too.

Although I didn't originate these principles, I work to implement them. While researchers are in their laboratories, my clients and I are walking the neighborhood hills or doing push-ups at the gym. But one thing is certain: No one can be successful in an exercise program unless he or she follows an exercise plan.

Training Basics

Actually, there's not that much to learn. There are only four variables in the design of your exercise program:

Type (mode of exercise)
Duration (length of the workout)
Frequency (how often you work out)
Intensity (how hard you work out)

These variables are applied to the aerobic phase of your one-hour exercise session. To progress and improve, I will change the variables and move you from one level of conditioning to the next. A **Duration** example is: You may start training with a 20-minute aerobic time and in six weeks extend that time to 26 minutes.

How To Find Your Training Heart Rate

To check your heart rate, you must take your pulse.

● Find your pulse. Use the index and middle finger only (the thumb has a pulse of its own). You can find your pulse on:

● The inside of the wrist, palm up, toward the thumb side of the wrist's center. A method professionals use, once the pulse point is determined, is to mark the spot with a pen to help find it quickly.

● The neck, about two inches in front of your ear and two inches lower than your jawbone. Place your fingers gently (pressing too hard slows the heart rate) on the large artery.

● If you have trouble finding the pulse point, walk around the room for 20 to 60 seconds and try again.

● It's easiest if you use a clock with a second hand or a digital readout. Begin counting with the next full beat starting with 0.

● Take a few practice counts for 10 seconds, and multiply them by 6 to determine the beats per minute.

● The 10-second count of heartbeats multiplied by six will be used whenever you check your training heart rate.

TYPE: What Exercise Activities Can I Use? Your program will emphasize aerobic exercise, which is so vital for overall health and weight control. An aerobic activity continuously and rhythmically uses the major-muscle groups of the body, primarily the legs. You get to move with aerobic exercise, which makes it a lot of fun. You can choose to walk (outdoors or on a treadmill), swim, cycle (outdoors or on a stationary bike), row (outdoors or on a rowing machine), run, cross-country ski (outdoors or on a machine), hike, or dance exercise.

Besides aerobic conditioning, your exercise plan will include stretches, calisthenics, and weight lifting. The aerobic activities also provide a measure of flexibility and strength.

DURATION: How Long Should I Exercise? How long you are able to work out is directly related to how intensely you work out. Obviously, the more moderate the activity, the longer you can continue it. And the longer you continue the aerobic segment, the more calories you'll burn. Depending on your level of fitness, the duration for the three types of exercise fits into your one-hour workout within these ranges.

Flexibility (warm-up) 5–10 minutes
Aerobic Exercise 20–31 minutes
Strength 14–24 minutes
Flexibility (cool-down) 5–10 minutes

FREQUENCY: How Often Do I Exercise? This is the part of the prescription that allows you to achieve your fitness goals. If you exercise too often, the body won't have enough time to rest and adapt to the stress of the exercises. If you don't exercise often enough, nothing will happen.

● **Aerobic** exercise can be done three to six times per week for a minimum of 20 continuous minutes. The maximum is six times per week.

● **Flexibility** exercises can be done six days a week.

● **Strength** exercises are best done three times per week when you work all the major-muscle groups at one time.

● **Rest** at least one day each week.

INTENSITY: How Hard Do I Exercise? Training at the correct intensity during exercise is probably the most essential factor in your exercise prescription. If you exercise too hard, you're asking for injuries and possible medical problems. It's a fast way to become an exercise dropout. And you may not get the results you desire despite the effort. On the other hand, you need to exercise hard enough to see and feel the results. The body's answer to the stress of exercise is adaptation. It adapts by stimulating the heart and lungs, muscles, tissues, and organs to become increasingly more efficient to handle the stress. "Overload" is what we call the stress we use to challenge the system so it will become stronger.

You can overload in several ways: by adding more time to the workout (extending the aerobic activity from 20 to 31 minutes); by gradually pushing your heart to work harder during aerobic activity; by adding repetitions (moving from ten to twenty-five sit-ups); or by using different exercises or weight during strength training to challenge the muscles in different ways.

To ensure that you are working at the appropriate intensity level during aerobic activity, you'll work in the **"training heart rate zone."** Your THR zone indicates a range of how hard your heart is working. The heart rate is measured by counting beats per minute. By exercising within your personalized heart rate zone, you'll get specific results, such as weight loss and increased aerobic capacity. It's unnecessary to count heartbeats during the stretching and strengthening activities because these activities do not use a continuous volume of oxygen.

You'll take your pulse for 10 seconds twice during the aerobic workout:

After **8 minutes** to make sure that you are increasing your heart rate.

After **15 minutes** to ensure that you are exercising in your personal training heart rate zone.

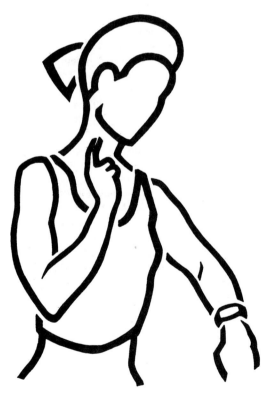

Find Your Pulse on the Wrist

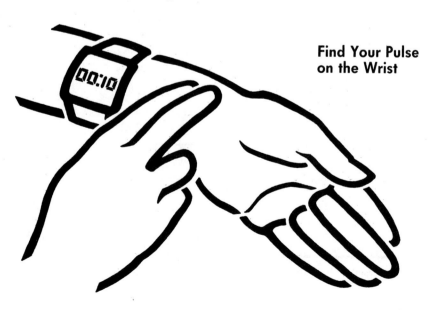

Find Your Pulse on the Neck

Using the Heart Rate Chart

The training heart rate zone defines the minimum and maximum number of heartbeats you should experience during exercise. It is expressed as a percentage of the maximum intensity you are capable of. By exercising within the *training heart rate zone*, you'll safely see results.

The most accurate method for determining the training zone that's right for you is the Karvonen formula (developed by M. J. Karvonen). It is the most accurate for each individual because it uses a measured or estimated maximum for your age, minus your resting heart rate.

You don't have to calculate your exercise heart rate. This has been done for you in the exercise heart rate chart at the right, which uses the Karvonen formula.

● To use the chart, you need to know your age and your resting heart rate. To find your resting heart rate, take your pulse before you climb out of bed for the next three mornings. Be prepared with a pen and paper on the nightstand. Count pulse beats for 30 seconds and multiply by two. Average the three readings.

● First, find your age on the chart, then locate the appropriate resting heart rate. Round off to the closest number. For example, if you are 32, your age on the chart is 30; if you are 36, go to 40. If your resting heart rate is 66, go to 70; if it's 74, go to 70.

● Second, find the program that you will be following. The heart rate range changes for each program.

● Third, based on the above information, locate your training heart rate zone. The top number (for example, 144–172) is the beats per minute. The bottom number (for example, 24–29) is the number of heart beats in the 10-second count. This number saves you time because you won't have to multiply by six each time.

Full Circle Fitness Heart Rate Chart

beats per minute—10-second count

Round Up to Nearest Age and Resting Heart Rate Age	(RPE Scale) Resting Heart Rate	(9–13) Gain 50–70%	(10–14) Train 55–75%	(11–15) Maintain 60–80%
20 years	60	130–158 22–26	137–165 23–28	144–172 24–29
	70	135–161 23–27	142–168 24–28	148–174 25–29
	80	140–164 23–27	146–170 24–28	152–176 25–29
30 years	60	125–151 21–25	132–158 22–26	138–164 23–27
	70	130–154 22–26	136–160 23–27	142–166 24–28
	80	135–157 23–26	140–162 23–27	146–168 24–28
40 years	60	120–144 20–24	126–150 21–25	132–156 22–26
	70	125–147 21–25	131–153 22–26	136–158 23–26
	80	130–150 22–25	135–155 23–26	140–160 23–27
50 years	60	115–137 19–23	121–143 20–24	126–148 21–25
	70	120–140 20–23	125–145 21–24	130–150 22–25
	80	125–143 21–24	130–148 22–25	134–152 22–25
60+ years	60	110–130 18–22	115–135 19–23	120–140 20–23
	70	115–133 19–22	120–138 20–23	124–142 21–24
	80	120–136 20–23	124–140 21–23	128–144 21–24

Perceived Exertion Scale

While counting heartbeats is a very effective method of assessing exercise intensity, it has two potential drawbacks. First, the heart rate ranges given on the chart are based on an estimate of the maximum heart rate for your age. While this is a good method when the maximum heart rate cannot actually be measured, it may not be right for you. Second, the amount of exertion you feel during exercise is a subjective measurement that may not compare with the objective measurement you get from counting heartbeats. For example, you may feel that you are working out too hard, even though you are working out in your training heart rate zone.

Because of this I would like to introduce a method of rating your exercise intensity based on what your perception of the effort is. It's very appropriately known as *The Rating of Perceived Exertion* (RPE). You will use a scale to identify a number that most accurately reflects how hard you feel you are working out during a given intensity of aerobic activity.

For example, walking very slowly on level ground would be perceived as being very, very light exertion by most people, while sprinting a long distance up a steep grade would eventually be perceived as very, very hard by anyone's standards.

With each program you will be given both a heart rate range and a perceived exertion range. You can use the perceived exertion to "double check" the heart rate range given on the chart. For example, if you choose *The Train Program* with the heart rate percentage of 55 to 75 percent, the intensity level for a 40-year old with a resting heart rate of 70 is either 131 to 153 beats per minute or 10 to 14 on the RPE scale, which is about "fairly light to hard."

If you are exercising at the heart rate range prescribed by the chart and the perception of the effort is less or greater than that recommended for your program, then adjust your heart rate range to stay within the prescribed perception of exertion.

6
7 Very, very light
8
9 Very light
10
11 Fairly light
12
13 Somewhat hard
14
15 Hard
16
17 Very hard
18
19 Very, very hard
20

Karvonen Formula Heart Rate	RPE Scale
Gain 50–70%	9–13
Train 55–75%	10–14
Maintain 60–80%	11–15
Handle on Health 60–80%	11–15
Competitive Edge 70–90%	12–16

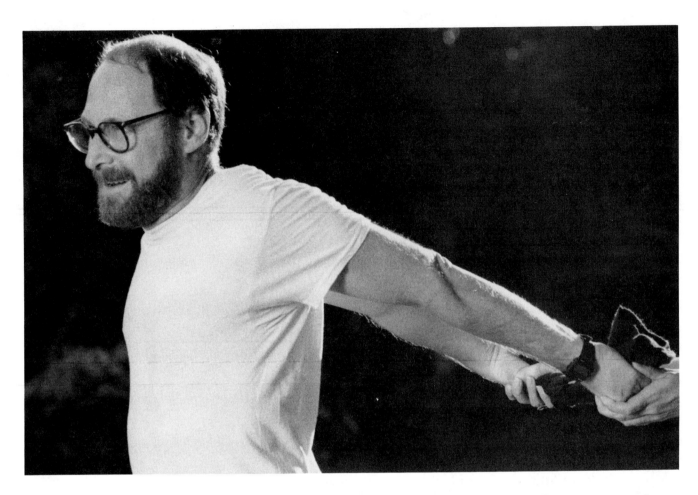

Exercise Progression

One of the most rewarding—and inspiring—aspects of exercise is watching the progress you make. But after you have achieved a basic foundation of fitness, or have adapted to a conditioning level, you'll have to change the variables in order to continue improving. As you move through the programs, each one has a little something different to offer to maintain the physical challenge and rekindle your interest. If, however, you wish to plateau your activity at any of the programs, you will still realize many of the health benefits of physical activity.

How long will it take to move through the programs? That depends a lot on how consistent you are and how well you master the activities.

Creating An Exercise Lifestyle

While I was doing the research for this book, I found a thought-provoking quote. It's a statement by P. O. Astrand, who's considered the father of exercise physiology. He said, "In principle, there is less risk in activity than continuous inactivity and it is more advisable to pass a careful medical examination if one intends to be sedentary in order to establish whether one's state of health is good enough to stand the inactivity."

Full Circle Fitness training programs start with a purposeful and planned three-hours-per-week commitment. But you can get more benefit from planned exercise by incorporating informal physical activity into your life *frequently*—every day. Create time with your family and friends being active, playing catch, or running after tennis balls—the little things add up!

"Fitness" is more than just exercise, although that's an important part of it. Your physical well-being is intricately interwoven with the mental and emotional aspects of your personality. When you are facing physical challenges, you are also facing nonphysical ones. It takes fortitude and courage to overcome time obstacles, to work out even when you're depressed or tired, to reduce alcohol and food intake, and to struggle past physical limitations. Friends and family are not always supportive of regular exercise, and old habits are hard to change.

The rewards of exercise are not strictly physical. I've already mentioned the stress release, mood elevation, increased concentration, and improved work performance that studies have shown accompany physical activity. The sense of accomplishment that overcoming obstacles brings can be a potent force in an individual's life, enabling a calm, good-humored outlook to emerge. And the increase in physical and mental energy can be quite surprising. More energy for fun with the family, for that special relationship, for personal accomplishment, or competitive sports.

Confronting and overcoming challenges builds internal strength while it teaches perspective, and perspective helps keep life balanced. For optimum fitness, mix regular exercise with time for family and work, a hobby or sport, and restful sleep. Although I am encouraging you to schedule time for exercise, don't become so obsessed with a plan or a specific goal that you burn out, and eventually drop out. Enjoy exercise as one of the many activities that make a happy and full life. Ultimately, physical activity is a key to knowing and renewing yourself.

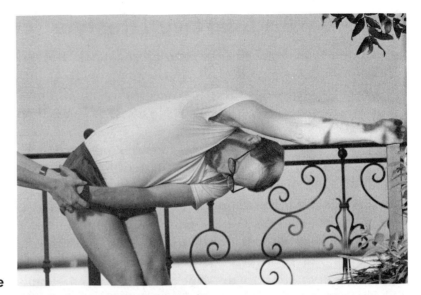

Flexibility Exercise

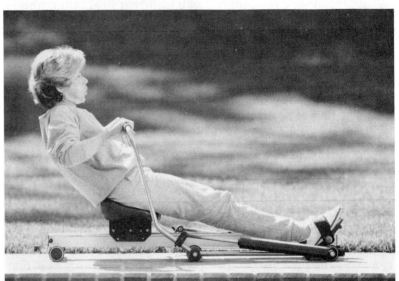

Aerobic Exercise

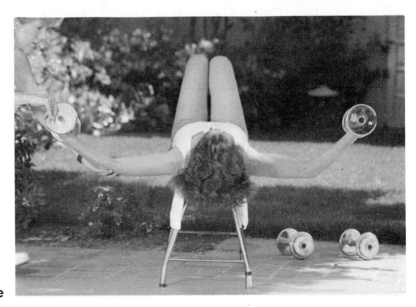

Strength Exercise

4

TRAINING SECRETS FOR SUCCESS

So far we've talked a lot about exercise and its benefits. Now it's time to meet the physical activities that comprise the one-hour workout session. While some people approach the exercises as if they're meeting unwelcome strangers, it's better to greet them as friends. You'll be spending a lot of time together!

In addition to the flexibility, strength, and aerobic exercises, you'll be introduced to a practical and effective eating plan in Chapter 10 that will help you maintain or control your weight and fuel an active lifestyle. The secret to health is balance, and it takes all of these elements to achieve whole-body results.

Whether you're a newcomer or an experienced exerciser, it will take several sessions for you to master the skills of the program you select. After you're familiar with the routines, the exercises will become much more fun. You can enjoy being more expert in your movements and begin to feel rhythm, control, and relaxation. As you advance, your exercise experience will allow you to determine the intensity of activity, diversify your routine, and utilize training techniques to achieve a personalized program that grows with you.

Know Your Muscles

These anatomical illustrations show the muscles we'll be exercising in the strength phase of your session. All *Full Circle Fitness* programs train the major muscle groups of the body, and the exercises you follow will "work" these muscles in a systematic order. What you do to one side of the body, you do to the other. By balancing the muscle groups, each program ensures equal gains in strength and flexibility, muscle size and shape, and prevents unnecessary muscle soreness or immobility.

   I want you to start thinking of your body in terms of the major muscle groups and how they work together: chest and upper back, shoulders and arms, abdominals and lower back, front and back of the legs. By keeping these groupings in mind, it helps you remember what muscle group to exercise and the order of the strength exercises.

   By establishing an order, you can

see the end of your workout at the beginning and what exercises you'll be doing to get there. The order ensures whole-body strength training and functions as a trainer would, so you can relax and concentrate on the specific muscle you are working.

   When you are doing an exercise to increase the strength or tone of a muscle, think of the goal number of times you want to try doing it. These are repetitions or reps. The repeat of that number after a rest is called sets. Though it may seem harder, repeating the same repetitions after a rest strengthens the muscle and gives it endurance.

   While it is natural to feel some discomfort and post-exercise soreness when you begin using muscles in challenging new ways, pain or extreme discomfort is a sign you're probably doing too much too soon. Slow down. By the way, it's common for tired muscles to remind you of your first exercise sessions. Curious but true, the best remedy for banishing soreness is one day of rest and more exercise!

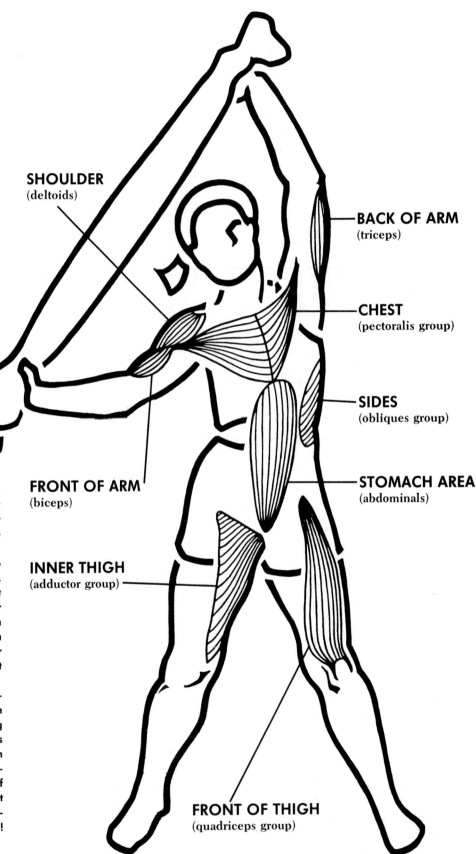

SHOULDER
(deltoids)

BACK OF ARM
(triceps)

CHEST
(pectoralis group)

SIDES
(obliques group)

STOMACH AREA
(abdominals)

FRONT OF ARM
(biceps)

INNER THIGH
(adductor group)

FRONT OF THIGH
(quadriceps group)

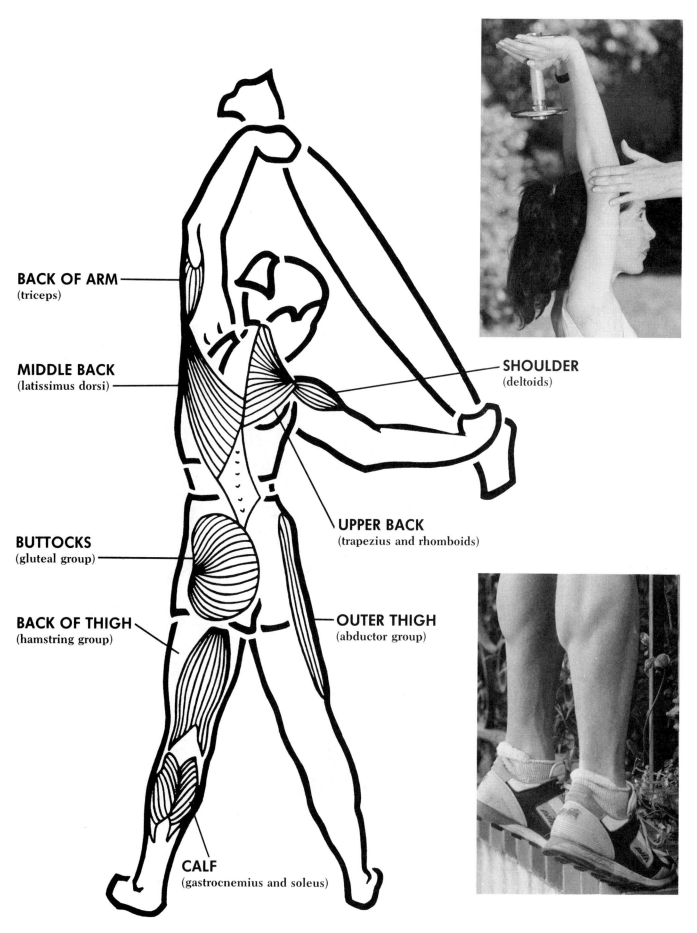

BACK OF ARM
(triceps)

MIDDLE BACK
(latissimus dorsi)

BUTTOCKS
(gluteal group)

BACK OF THIGH
(hamstring group)

CALF
(gastrocnemius and soleus)

SHOULDER
(deltoids)

UPPER BACK
(trapezius and rhomboids)

OUTER THIGH
(abductor group)

A Flexibility Routine

This unique style of stretching is designed to move from one exercise to the next, with minor adjustments between positions. You do not start and stop, but keep a continuous flow of movement, working one side of the body at a time. This creates a full-body flexibility routine that can be memorized.

Stretches are used at the beginning of every exercise session to gently prepare your muscles and heart for the aerobic conditioning that will follow. Each exercise in your routine will highlight the muscle group being used so you

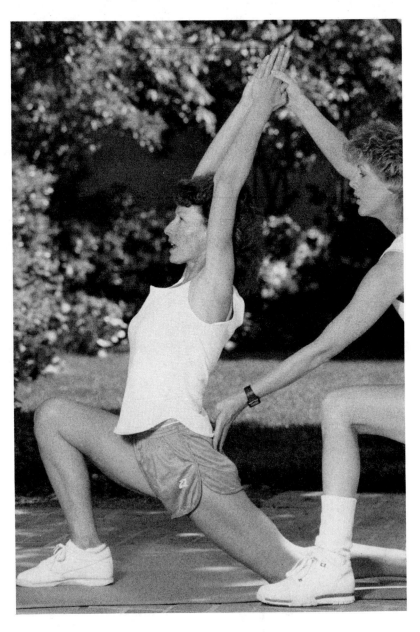

know what muscles you are stretching. For a cool-down at the end of the hour, the remaining stretches will relax your muscles to help prevent soreness, stiffness, and injury.

No matter how inflexible you are today, you can become more limber over a period of time if you keep stretching consistently and correctly. Remember that flexibility training is completely noncompetitive. Don't try to outstretch your partner or strain to touch toes that feel as if they're a mile away.

Secrets of Stretching

Warm up your muscles before stretching. If you train early in the morning or during cold weather, I suggest you jog in place for a few minutes to increase blood flow and raise muscle temperature before you begin stretching. If you are working out later in the day, it is not as necessary to jog before your training session.

Exhale as you stretch and inhale as you move into the next position. Breathing properly will help you stretch correctly and effectively. Exhaling on the stretch enables you to relax the muscle to its maximum length. Controlled breathing facilitates an unhurried pace.

Stretch until you feel tension, then hold the position for 10 to 30 seconds. Holding the position 10 to 30 seconds gives the muscle time to respond by relaxing and lengthening. Pay attention to the tension in the muscle in each position: Ease up if you feel sudden pain or extreme discomfort in the muscle that's stretching. Don't stretch beyond the point where you have complete control over the movement.

Do not bounce to gain flexibility. Never thrust your body weight in a bouncing movement in the attempt to maximize a stretch. It won't help your flexibility because bouncing doesn't *stretch* the muscles, and the bouncing could tear muscle fibers.

Be precise when moving into position. Concentration and control are flexibility skills that allow you to stretch your muscles properly because the position and movement of every part of your body is interrelated. For example, the placement of the foot and turn of the leg will affect the position of your back.

Move smoothly and leisurely and *breathe*. The transition between positions should not be awkward. Continual slow exhalation through the mouth and steady inhalation through the nose helps to keep the movements flowing and smooth.

Maximizing Aerobic Exercise

This portion of your exercise prescription can be a lot of fun because there are plenty of aerobic options to choose from. Which ones will you do regularly? Let your personal preferences—whether to row or bike or jog—be the deciding factor. Doing what you like will help you exercise consistently so you can condition your heart and lungs, control your weight, modify the risk of disease, and elevate your spirits.

Like other exercisers, you'll profit from alternating among many aerobic activities. Cross-training, as this approach is called, is a great way to maintain your interest, exercise different muscle groups for improved fitness, and prevent overuse injuries. I suggest you switch activities according to:

Time—alternate activities weekly, monthly, or daily: cycling with walking; swimming with running;

Seasons—cross-country ski in the winter and swim in the summer.

Before you select an aerobic activity, seriously examine your time schedule, lifestyle, and location. Bad weather, early darkness, and poor air quality are a few reasons to exercise indoors. If your realistic appraisal indicates you'd spend more time in your home than outside it, invest in one of the exercise machines that are described. If you'll use it, then it's practical and worth every penny.

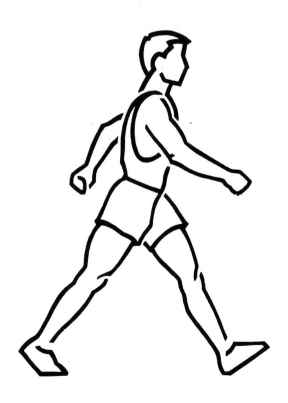

Aerobic Training Tips

Monitor your exercise intensity twice during each aerobic workout. The intensity level determines the value of aerobic exercise, so take your pulse at 8 minutes and 15 minutes into the activity to make sure you are within your training heart rate zone. Pay attention to the RPE scale. Adjust your heart rate to stay within the perceived exertion range recommended for your program.

Take the time to learn the proper form and method for each activity. There is a correct technique and posture for all these activities. Moving correctly prevents injuries and optimizes the benefit of the exercise.

Move continuously for at least 20 minutes. If you stop and start or cut short the exercise session, you won't derive the benefits of aerobic exercise. In the beginning, you may be unable to work out that long. Go as long as you can, then walk briskly to complete the 20-minute minimum.

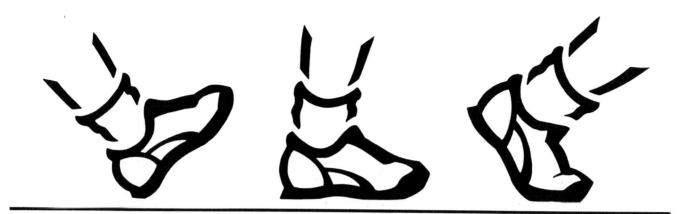

If you exercise outdoors, accommodate to the weather. During very hot weather, aerobic exercisers can overheat, which may lead to sunstroke or heat prostration. Don't exercise outdoors during the middle of the day (between 11:30 A.M–2:30 P.M.), in very hot weather, or when the air is very polluted. Choose another activity you can do indoors or do the aerobic phase on another day.

In cold weather, keep your muscles warm with adequate layers of clothing, and when it's 20 degrees or less, either make sure you are properly dressed or exercise indoors.

Seven Aerobic Exercises to Explore

Walking Walking is an activity for everyone regardless of age, weight, or fitness level. Because it does not place excess strain on the legs and feet, walkers can avoid injuries while improving their conditioning levels.

A good walking pace covers one mile in 12 to 20 minutes depending on your age and fitness level. To work up to a challenging pace, alternate brisk walking with slow walking, keeping your heart rate elevated in the training heart rate zone.

Once you improve after at least four weeks of training, you will have to walk faster or add hills to reach your training heart rate zone.

Lead with your heel and roll onto the ball of your foot as you swing your arms in opposition to the feet and stride forward. Your legs should swing freely from the hip sockets with knees relaxed and slightly bent. Be aware of your posture and keep the rib cage in line with the hip bone. Lean forward about 5 degrees as you stride with a smooth motion. Breathe normally.

Shoes For Walking

Shoes are the most important piece of equipment for walking. There needs to be sufficient cushioning to minimize impact of the stride and reduce injury to the foot. Fit is critical, so try on several pairs before choosing. Quality of construction is a stronger consideration than price. Be careful that the heel wedge does not aggravate pronation (foot rolls inward) of the foot. Consistent use (twenty miles a week) will wear down the cushioning material, so check the condition of yours about every three to four months. If you are experiencing foot, shin, or knee difficulties from walking, consult an orthopedist or podiatrist, and take along your shoes.

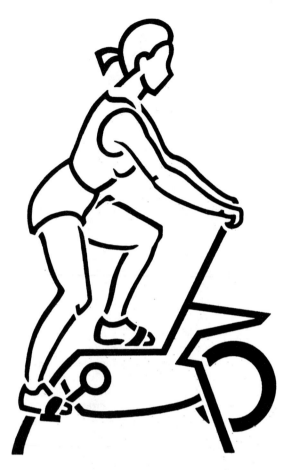

For indoors, a stationary bicycle should have a solid front flywheel or fan, an adjustable seat, and a reliable method of controlling resistance on the flywheel. I particularly prefer bikes that actually measure the workload on a gauge.

Cycling Whether you ride outside with the wind in your face or indoors while watching the news, cycling is a low-stress exercise. It is excellent for beginning exercisers or those with orthopedic problems because the seat supports a lot of the body's weight. Be sure the seat height is adjusted so that the knee is bent slightly when the pedal is closest to the ground. Beware of long pants that can get caught in the chain.

Intensity is determined by how fast you are pedaling and by the amount of resistance on the wheel (indoor) or the percentage of grade (outdoor). Once you are conditioned you will have to increase speed or pedal against more resistance to maintain your training heart rate zone.

Indoor Cycling On a stationary exercise bike, an adjustable resistance control can progressively increase the workload. As you increase the load on the flywheel, or pedal faster, you will notice your heart rate responds to the higher intensity of work. The speedometer helps you to keep a steady rhythm or cadence. To warm up during the first 3 minutes of cycling, be sure to ride at a steady pace at low resistance or pedal rate of approximately 50–70 revolutions per minute.

Outdoor Cycling Posture differs depending on whether you are using dropped or upright handlebars. I prefer upright handlebars for recreational riding and for those with low-back discomfort. Thoroughly research cycling equipment and the proper technique for your specific cycle. If you are not riding on a measured course, attach an odometer to the cycle to monitor your distance. There are some slick electronic ones that measure time, distance, and pedal rate. For outdoor cycling, always wear a light-weight, well-made, protective helmet with a chin strap.

Swimming A terrific workout for the whole body, the water's resistance conditions the muscles while stimulating the heart for aerobic conditioning. Because water also supports the weight of the body, swimming doesn't stress the tendons, ligaments, and joints, which is why it's the aerobic exercise of choice for rehabilitating injuries.

Intensity Studies have shown that swimming does not raise your heart rate as high as upright exercise does for the same duration and amount of work. In a prone position your heart does not work as hard against gravity and is able to pump more blood with each beat. To calculate your training heart rate range while swimming, use the Karvonen heart rate chart in Chapter 3 and subtract 12 beats from the one-minute training heart rate or subtract 2 beats when you count your pulse beats for 10 seconds. By staying within the recommended range for perceived exertion your heart rate will be less than upright exercise.

If you are just taking up swimming as regular exercise, I suggest enrolling in a swim program to refine your technique. Awkward swimming strokes or improper breathing will tire you quickly and reduce the benefits of the exercise.

If you swim continuous laps regularly, try varying your swim routine with:

Interval swims—change the length of each interval or the duration of rest periods between them.

Pyramid laps—increase the number of laps broken with a rest period until you reach a goal number of repetitions (one lap, rest—two laps, rest—three laps, rest—) to the set goal, then work down with intermittent rests (five laps, rest—four laps, rest—three laps, rest—etc.) back to the finish.

The ideal water temperature is about 75 to 80 degrees Fahrenheit; any warmer than that and you cannot dissipate the heat created by the exercise. Swim coaches generally recommend that beginners start in a 20- to 25-meter pool and progress to the 50-meter Olympic size. Smaller pools require frequent turning, which reduces the intensity level. Pools with gutters, lane buoys, or painted lines on the bottom guide your path. You may have to wear a swim watch with a second hand or digital readout if there is no clock at the pool.

If you swim in a public pool, you'll need goggles and a swim cap. Lycra suits are supportive and fit snugly, and racing straps will keep the suit on you. When you want a swimming challenge and more fun, try a kickboard, pull buoy, or hand paddles.

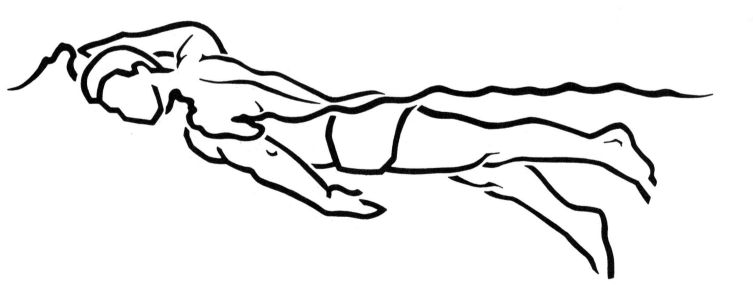

Cross-Country Skiing Cross-country skiing enables the heart to pump more blood to the arms, legs, and trunk than any other exercise can. Although it is among the most demanding of endurance activities, cross-country skiing is also one of the most effortless once you learn the skills. It feels easy because the push-and-glide motion is impact-free, which also makes it a good exercise for a person with knee problems.

Indoor Cross-Country A great indoor workout is a cross-country ski machine for improving and maintaining your aerobic capacity as well as your ski technique. Using ropes or handles instead of poles, the indoor equivalent can be just as invigorating as the real thing. The push-glide motion is a little different in that you are unable to move forward. Moving your arms and legs in opposition is a great workout for hips, legs, abdomen, and buttocks as well as your heart.

A machine that uses foot pillows and long poles is often easiest to begin with if you've never cross-country skied. If you're an experienced skier, graduate to a model with simulated skis and ropes.

Outdoor Cross-Country Coordinating the arms and legs does take some practice, but you can learn the fundamentals in a weekend. Besides, winter scenery is so inviting, you'll be skiing for winters to come. I recommend exercising with a partner while learning the motion.

For super skiers, telemarking, which is like hiking on skis, has become very popular. There are no limits to where you can venture or explore. Acquire the skills before you apply this or any new sport to your aerobic program.

A rental store can provide the skis, poles, bindings, and boots. Winter sun and snow are fun, but you must wear goggles and sunscreen for protection against burn and snow blindness.

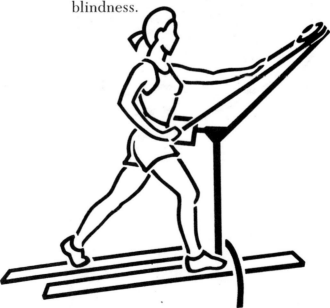

Cross-Country Ski Machine

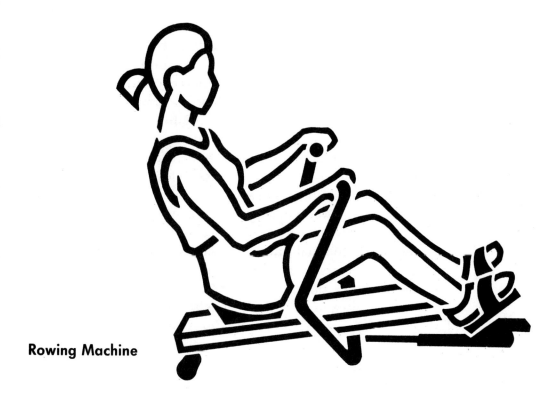

Rowing Machine

Rowing An excellent aerobic conditioner because it uses so many muscles, rowing minimizes injuries by eliminating impact on the body. Since it uses resistance, rowing improves muscle strength as well as endurance.

Indoor Rowing There are varieties of rowing machines available that use different methods to create resistance. There are two basic types of designs, the flywheel and the piston. On a flywheel machine you work against a braking force of wind resistance, friction, or electric resistance. This design feels most like real rowing because it has a continuous momentum that approximates gliding.

For convenience and compactness, the piston design works quite well. The resistance is created by the pistons as you pull back with your arms, push with your legs, and slide back on the seat. Although you are using your arms, your legs do a lot of the work. To make rowing harder, simply increase the resistance or row faster. Many machines come with digital readouts that count strokes per minute and total strokes, and a clock that measures the time you've been rowing. If you have a bad back or heart trouble, check with your doctor before rowing.

Outdoor Rowing On a lake, bay, or river, rowing is a lot of fun, which makes it easy to keep up for a period of time. Since it requires specialized equipment, it's best to locate a rowing coach to explain the available craft and oars and provide instruction.

Low- and Mixed-Impact Dance Exercise A unique advantage of aerobic dance exercise is its ability to exercise the entire body with gains in flexibility, coordination, and agility. Another is the music, which is motivating, fun, and helpful for maintaining an appropriate intensity level.

Low- and mixed-impact dance exercise minimizes the classic jumps and hops of aerobic dancing by utilizing more arm movements and keeping feet close to the ground. A well-conditioned person may add one-half pound hand or wrist weights to intensify the workout.

The intensity level of dance exercise depends a great deal on individual effort, so remember to take your pulse regularly to assure you are achieving the appropriate training heart rate range.

Many exercise studios, health clubs, businesses, and locally sponsored projects offer instructor-led classes in dance exercise. Make sure the instructor is willing to answer questions, chooses safe exercises, and is qualified to instruct.

You can also make up your own routine to a home-made music tape that has eight-beat rhythmic music. Position slower tempos at the beginning for warm-up and the end for cool-down. Change the routines regularly to maintain your interest. Or, read announcements of commercial tapes and choose one that is recommended by a knowledgeable reviewer.

Well-cushioned aerobics shoes that provide foot stability are important. Running shoes will not work for the lateral movements of dance exercise. Aerobics shoes will need to be replaced about every three to four months because of the breakdown of the cushioning material.

Jogging/Running You can run almost anywhere—on a track, through city streets and parks, down rural roadways, or in your living room—which makes its convenience a big plus.

If you have been inactive, begin by walking. As your conditioning level improves, insert short stretches of jogging into your workouts. Lengthen these segments until you're completely on the run.

The length of time you jog or run is more important than the number of miles you cover. Stay within your target heart rate zone and pay attention to your perceived exertion. If you can carry on a conversation while running, you are probably training at the proper intensity. As you improve, add 10 percent of the total time you run to determine the following week's goal. Be sure to follow this formula and don't try to do too much too soon.

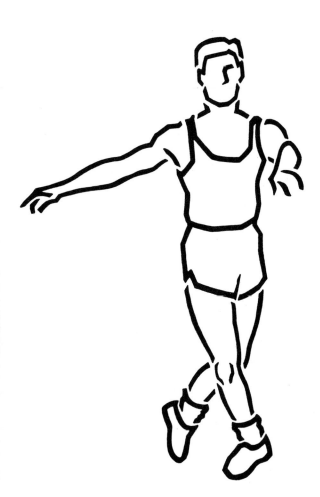

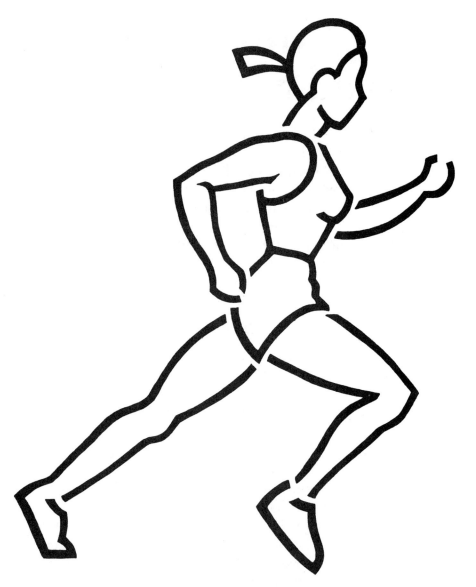

Example: If your total running time is 30 minutes for a session, then add only 3 minutes a week. This will allow you to build your endurance over time while minimizing your chance of injuries.

Equally important is observing good running form, which increases the efficiency of the activity by reducing jarring up-and-down motions. Developing a natural fluid style not only helps you avoid injury, but allows you to realize running's potential as a superb conditioner.

Running shoes should be well-cushioned and supportive as well as lightweight. Shoes that are overly worn can lead to injuries, so replace them as soon as the cushioning material breaks down, approximately every three to four months for regular runners. A thicker tread is utilitarian for slick, snowy, or icy streets. On a track, a thinner tread will allow you to run faster. If you run after dark, reflective clothing can prevent an accident.

Muscle Endurance and Strength Training

During the strength portion of your workout, it helps to apply your mental muscle. The power, physical beauty, and strength benefits of muscle training are optimized when you concentrate on what you're doing.

To challenge your muscles, you'll create resistance with your own body (as with push-ups) and with dumbbells. Since there are different strength exercises for each program you'll find the resistance routine geared for you personally. Be sure to review these guidelines before you begin training.

Strength Training Secrets

Move from large-muscle groups to smaller ones. For example, begin with the chest (pectoralis group) and finish with the arms (biceps/triceps).

Exercise one side of the body, then exercise the opposing muscle group. For instance, follow the front of the arm (biceps) with the back of the arm (triceps).

Push, then pull. After you push with one muscle group, then pull with the opposing group. You push with your chest and pull with your back.

It is important to understand the execution of each exercise. Correct form is a must for effectiveness and safety. Check your body's position at the starting point, through the path of motion, and at completion. Try several slow-motion dry runs of each exercise from the beginning through the end.

Close your eyes, concentrate, and use your "mind's eye" to focus on, or isolate, the muscles you are using. By paying mental attention to the sequence and form, you can move accurately and confidently. Proper form will place stress on the muscles you intend to work and not on muscles that happen to be in the vicinity.

Exhale on the contraction—the lift or push—and inhale during the extension or opposite movement. Don't hold your breath. It is important to utilize the return trip of each exercise because it works the muscle as much as the contraction does, but in a different way.

Use slow, fully controlled movements in both directions without permitting momentum to do any of the work. Uncontrolled fast motions do not exercise the muscles, and invite injury.

Move through the complete range of motion that you can achieve. Your muscles do not develop fully when motion is incomplete.

Use the suggested resistance or weight for each program. Too little or too much resistance won't gradually overload. Work the maximum repetitions for three sets in your program before you start increasing weight.

Record Your Workout

The extensive written records I keep of every client allow both of us to be absolutely sure about what happened at the previous session and what is needed to maintain progress. It's fun to look back and compare progress from two sets of five push-ups to fifteen in a matter of weeks. Training notes can be invaluable for you, too, as long as you immediately record the exercises so you don't forget them. Take notes as you go along. It's amazing how quickly you can forget the details. Written records are especially valuable for strength training because repetitions and pounds continually change as you improve. It's difficult to remember exactly which exercises you performed and how much resistance was used without keeping notes on each session. See the Appendix for all the information you need to create your own workout book.

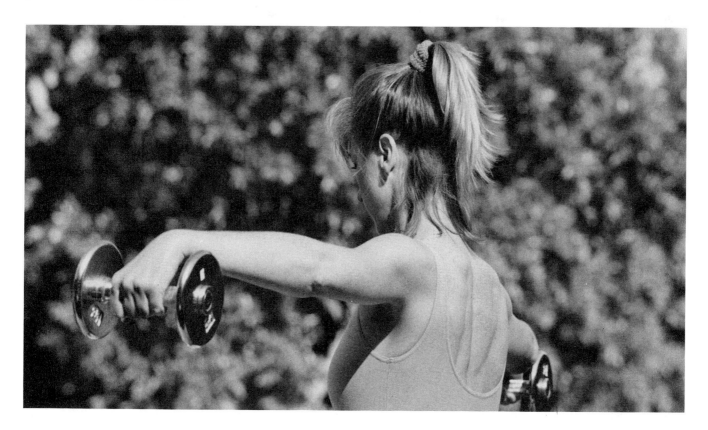

5

If you haven't exercised regularly for the past six months, are fifteen pounds or more overweight, scored low in the fitness assessments, then this is the program to get you moving for the next six weeks.

THE GAIN PROGRAM

Everyone makes resolutions to exercise, but how many people are actually doing it after three months? Not many. However, once you've made a resolution, *The Gain Program* will get you started and help you to build an exercise routine that you can easily follow.

With this program you'll become more aware of your body, start to burn fat, and have equal time dedicated to aerobic, strength, and flexibility training. That's important because as the heart and lungs improve it's necessary to stretch and strengthen the muscles, ligaments, and tendons. The combination of these three components prepares the body for a future of regular exercise that will show obvious results and minimize injuries.

It will take you six months to move through the Gain, Train, and Maintain programs, so stay with the order and program requirements as listed below. The key to this plan is to get started today. That's right, just get to your planned session and the results will unfold.

Training Tips For The Gain Program

Before you begin, step outside of yourself and survey your physical situation objectively. *You* are not fat, although your body may be. It's not at all easy to be objective, but you have to learn to stop identifying with the "bad"

THE COMPETITIVE EDGE OR **A HANDLE ON HEALTH**

6 months and on

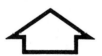

MAINTAIN
12 weeks

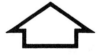

TRAIN
6 weeks

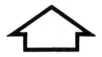

GAIN
6 weeks

and begin concentrating on your power to change for the better. It's when you berate yourself for imperfection that you start eating more ice cream.

Have a clock in sight while you exercise so that you keep to the schedule and don't get interrupted. If you're constantly being interrupted, you won't see results.

Keep to three workouts a week and that's all. When you take on too much, you're more likely to drop out.

Recognize that you will not see a "fantasy" you in the first three months. But you *can* start losing weight and feeling good in that period of time.

Keep a positive attitude. Remind yourself that you can make time for exercise, you can be healthy and in charge of your life. Take the time to enjoy yourself being active.

Work out with a partner. Have a companion help to keep your motivation high, your exercise appointments on schedule, and to have a second pair of eyes watching for correct execution of exercises.

Find unsuspected exercise areas and equipment in your home. Walls, steps, gates, or a bench can all be used for workouts.

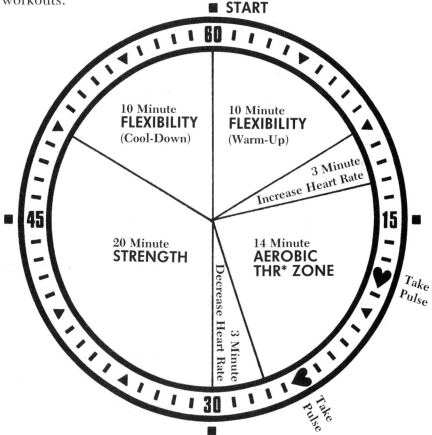

The Gain Exercise Hour
1 Hour Workout 3 Times per Week

Warm-Up Stretches

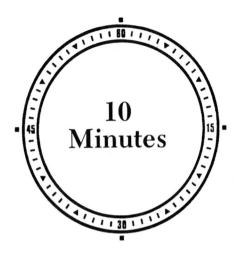

10 Minutes

Equipment

A mat or folded quilt and old bath towel.

Secrets of Stretching

● Warm up your muscles before stretching.
● Exhale as you stretch and inhale as you move into the next position.
● Stretch until you feel tension, then hold the position for 10 to 30 seconds.
● Avoid bouncing.
● Be precise when moving into position.
● Move smoothly and leisurely and *breathe*.
● Perform the stretches in the order listed.

Lower Body

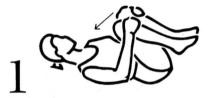

1 **THE TORTOISE** (for lower back) Lie on your back on the exercise mat and lift knees toward the chest with hands grasping the lower leg beneath the knee. Lengthen your neck and look straight up. Inhale through the nose and exhale through the mouth.
● Transition: Stay in the same position.

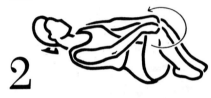

2 **KNEE CIRCLES** (for lower back) Slide your hands onto kneecaps and circle knees to the right 4 times, keeping abdominals pressed into the lower back so that the base of the spine is against the mat. Gradually make the circles smaller, then reverse the direction for 4 more circles, gradually making the circles larger.
● Transition: Keep one leg toward your chest and extend the other leg straight out along the mat, with the foot flexed so your toes point to the ceiling.

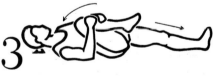

3 **THIGH TO CHEST** (for lower back) With hands clasped below the knee of the bent leg, exhale as you pull the thigh up and back toward your shoulder. Don't push down toward the ground, but gently pull in an arc toward the shoulder.
● Transition: Keep thigh in the same position, with the other leg still stretched out.

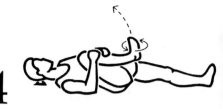

4 **FOOT CIRCLES** (for ankle) Circle the ankle of the bent leg 4 times to the right, than 4 times to the left.
● Transition: Place the foot of this leg on the knee of your outstretched leg.

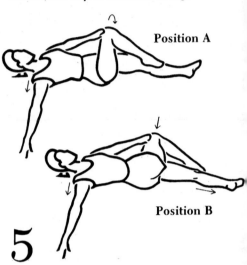

Position A

Position B

5 **BACK TWIST** (for back) Grasp the outside of the bent knee with the opposite hand. Stretch the other hand away from the body, level with the shoulder. Gently push the bent leg toward the floor while keeping your shoulders square on the mat. Exhale as you gently press downward, and inhale as you hold the stretch for at least 30 seconds. Use 3 or more exhalations to relax the leg toward the floor. Finally, turn your head away from the direction of the twist.
● Transition: Release the stretch and straighten your head.

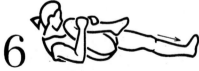

6 **KNEE TOUCH** (for back) With both hands, grasp beneath the knee. Lift your head, neck, and upper back from the floor and touch your kneecap with your nose.
● Transition: Return your head, upper body, and bent leg to the mat.

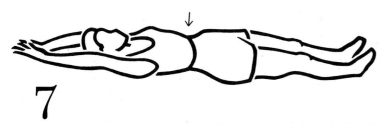

7

FULL-BODY STRETCH (for all major muscles) Stretch your arms overhead and extend both legs as you exhale. Press abdominals toward the floor to keep lower back flat.
● Transition: Roll onto your stomach, bringing arms to the side of the hips.

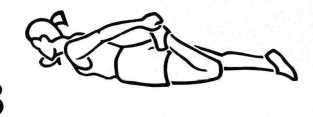

8

THIGH PULL (for top of thigh) Lying on your stomach, take hold of the foot with the hand on the same side of the body and pull the lower leg and foot to the buttocks.
● Transition: Release your grasp on the foot and place both hands under the shoulders with forearms flat on the floor, and head looking down at the mat.

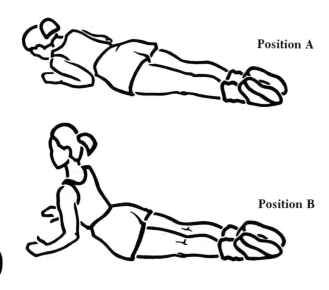

Position A

Position B

9

COBRA (for back and abdominals) Pressing the palms of the hands into the floor lift the upper body without collapsing the shoulders, using the bent forearms to raise the torso while pelvis remains on the floor.
● Transition: Lower your torso until you are flat on the mat. Push yourself up until you are sitting on knees and feet.

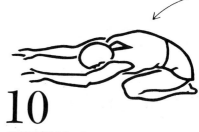

10

SLEEPING CAT (for lower back) Exhale as you bend from the waist and extend your arms out in front of you until your chest is on your thighs.
● First Transition: Roll onto your back and start series with *Thigh to Chest* on the other side.
● Second Transition: After completing the series on the opposite side through the *Sleeping Cat*, raise your torso and sit on your heels.

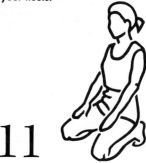

11

TOE CURL (for arches of feet) Distribute your weight evenly as you sit on your heels with toes pressed forward underneath you. Inhale as you press through your arches. Place hands on thighs and straighten your back as you exhale.
● Transition: Relax toes so that tops of your feet are against the mat. Sit on your heels and shift weight to your knees.

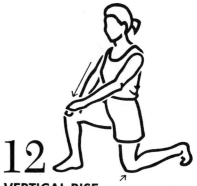

12

VERTICAL RISE (to protect back upon standing) Bring one foot forward so that your thigh parallels the floor. Place both hands on top of the knee in front of you, and pull the toes of your rear foot forward. Press down on the knee, stabilizing your balance as you stand up.

Warm-Up Stretches Continue

Warm-Up Stretches

Upper Body

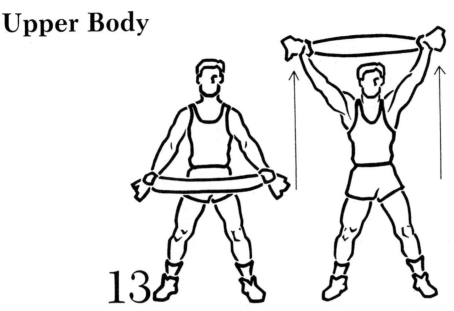

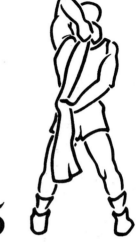

13

SHOULDER ARCH (for shoulders) Taking the towel in both hands, stand with your feet farther than shoulder-width apart with arms straight. Without locking your elbows, raise both your arms in an arc, keeping the towel taut, until hands swing behind the head. Lower your hands to the thighs and repeat the movement smoothly 5 times.
● Transition: Hold the last stretch above the head and bend the knees slightly.

15

ARM PULL (for back of arm) Bring your free arm behind your back to grab the towel at a comfortable distance. The arm holding the towel should be near the ear with the elbow pointing forward. Pull down on the towel to stretch the back of the bent arm as you exhale. Hold the stretch for 3 deep breaths, keeping the tension in the towel constant. Then switch the towel to the other hand and repeat the stretch.
● Transition: Let go of the towel with the upper arm and extend both arms downward with palms facing toward the rear. Grasp both ends and stretch the towel behind your back.

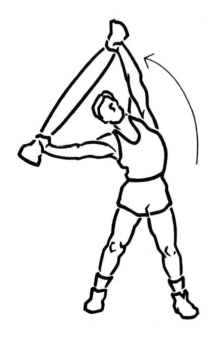

14

SIDE STRETCH (for sides of the trunk) Keeping the towel taut, exhale as you use one hand to pull the towel downward, bending the trunk to one side. Prevent your back from arching by tightening the abdominal muscles. Increase the stretch for 3 deep breaths by pulling down on the towel with the lower arm, continuing to bend to the side. Slowly stand straight and repeat the stretch on the opposite side.
● Transition: Stand erect, knees slightly bent, towel over head. Bend your elbows and release your grip from one end of the towel so the towel is hanging to the floor behind you.

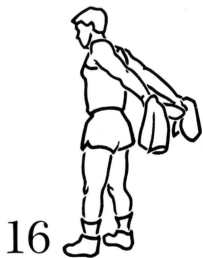

16

CHEST PULL (for chest) Holding the towel in a straight line, lift both arms straight up until you feel the stretch in the chest and shoulder muscles. Take 3 deep breaths in this position while the muscles relax.

Aerobic Conditioning

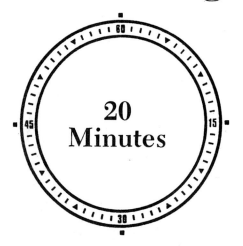

Activity Walk, stationary cycle, rowing machine, low-impact dance exercise (beginning level). Combine these if you are unable to do one activity for 20 minutes: for example, cycle and walk.

Intensity **3 minutes** to elevate heart rate—**14 minutes** in your personal heart rate zone—**3 minutes** to decrease heart rate to 100–110 beats per minute

The Gain Heart Rate Chart

Round Up to Nearest Age and Resting Heart Rate		(RPE Scale) 9–13	
Age	Resting Heart Rate		Gain 50–70%
	60		130–158
			22–26
20 years	70		135–161
			23–27
	80		140–164
			23–27
	60		125–151
			21–25
30 years	70		130–154
			22–26
	80		135–157
			23–26
	60		120–144
			20–24
40 years	70		125–147
			21–25
	80		130–150
			22–25
	60		115–137
			19–23
50 years	70		120–140
			20–23
	80		125–143
			21–24
	60		110–130
			18–22
60+ years	70		115–133
			19–22
	80		120–136
			20–23

beats per minute—10-second count

Aerobic Training Tips

● Monitor your exercise intensity twice during each aerobic workout: Take your pulse at 8 minutes and 15 minutes into the activity.
● Take the time to learn the proper form and method for each activity.
● Move continuously for at least 20 minutes.
● If you exercise outdoors, accommodate to the weather.

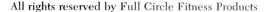

Strength Training

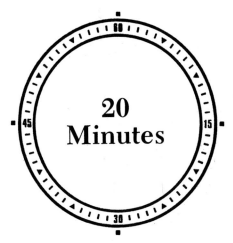

20 Minutes

Equipment

- 3–5-pound dumbbells for women
- 5–8-pound dumbbells for men
- "Record Your Workout" chart

Strength Training Secrets

- It is important to understand the execution of each exercise.
- Close your eyes, concentrate, and use your "mind's eye" to focus on, or isolate, the muscles you are using.
- Exhale on the contraction—the lift or push—and inhale during the opposite movement.
- Use slow, fully controlled movements in both directions without permitting momentum to do any of the work.
- Move through the complete range of motion that you can achieve.
- Sets are a defined number of repetitions (reps) done consecutively (i.e., 1–2 sets, or times).
- Use the suggested resistance or weight for each program.
- Keep exercises in the indicated sequence.

The Gain Program

CHEST
1. **Wall Push-aways**, 8 reps × 2 sets
or
1. **Incline Push-ups**, 8 reps × 2 sets

BACK
1. **One-Arm Rows**, dumbbells, 8 reps × 2 sets (each side)

SHOULDERS
1. **Pouring the Water**, dumbbells, 8 reps × 2 sets
2. **Straight Arm Raises**, dumbbells, 8 reps × 2 sets

ARMS
1. **Concentration Curls**, dumbbells, 8 reps × 2 sets
2. **Kickbacks**, dumbbells, 8 reps × 2 sets (each side)

ABDOMINALS
1. **Curl-ups**, 8 reps × 2 sets
2. **Crunches**, 8 reps × 2 sets
3. **One Leg Lift and Twist**, 8 reps × 2 sets (each side)

LEGS
1. **Leg Circles**, 8 forward and 8 backward (each leg)
2. **Outer Thigh Lifts**, 24 reps × 1 set (each leg)
3. **Inner Thigh Lifts**, 24 reps × 1 set (each leg)
or
1. **Lunge Walks**, 16 reps × 1 set
2. **Calf Raises**, 16 reps × 1 set

You have a choice of exercises.
Refer to your strength program chart.

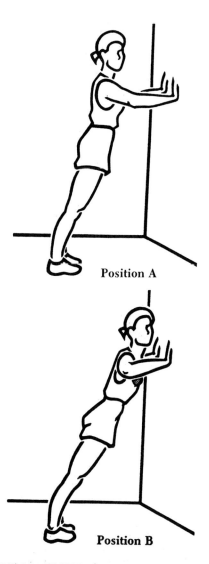

Position A

Position B

WALL PUSH-AWAYS Stand an arm's length away from a wall with hands at chest level, palms flat on the wall, fingertips toward the ceiling. Move your feet one or two steps farther away from the wall. Contract your stomach muscles. Inhale as you move your body, in one unit, toward the wall (head to the side), letting your elbows move to the sides. Exhale as you push away.

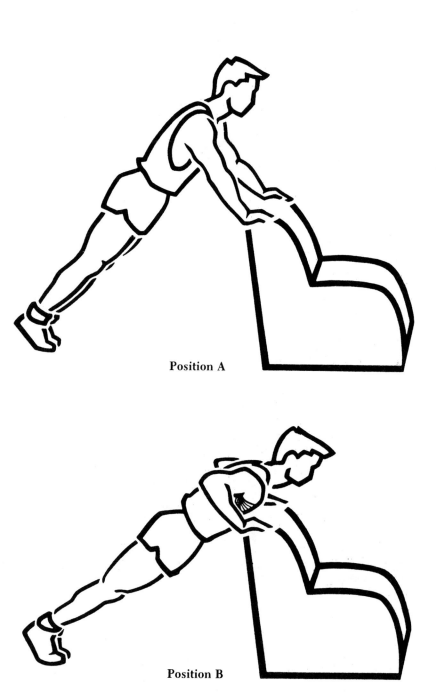

Position A

Position B

INCLINE PUSH-UPS Stand an arm's length away from a low bench, couch, or other sturdy surface with hands shoulder-width apart. Take one or two steps farther back. Keep your body straight in one line from the top of your head to your heels, with heels raised. Support your back by contracting the abdominal muscles. As your elbows go out to the side, lower your chest to the bench while you inhale. Then exhale as you press your body away.

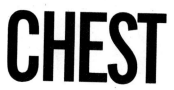

CHEST

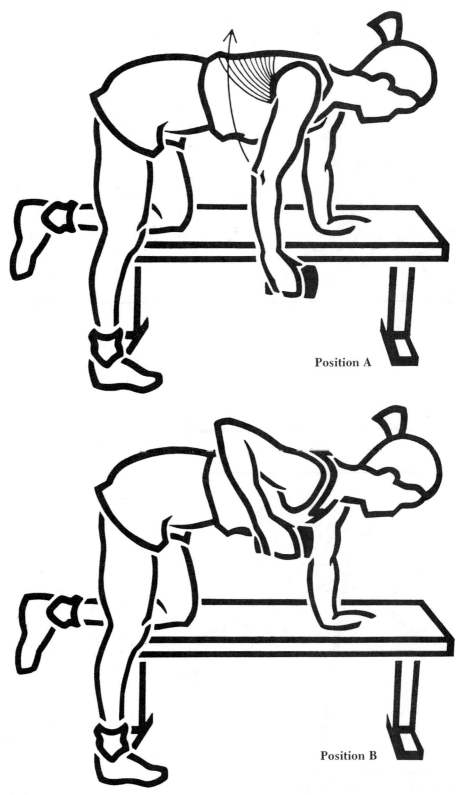

Position A

Position B

BACK

ONE-ARM ROWS Rest the arm and leg of one side on a low bench holding a dumbbell in the free hand. Keeping your shoulder immobile and your back flat, raise the weight straight up along the side of your body to just below the armpit. Exhale as you lift the bell, inhale as you lower it.

Position A

Position B

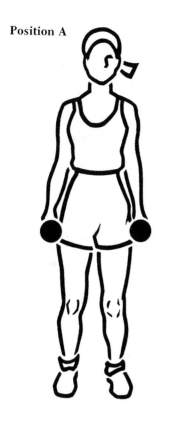
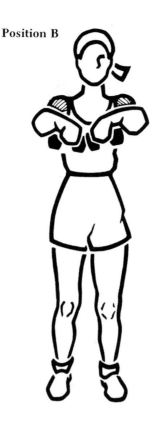

POURING THE WATER Stand tall with shoulders relaxed, hands at your side holding dumbbells, knees relaxed and feet about shoulder-width apart. Exhale as you raise your hands to chest level, palms down, and turn your hands slightly as if you're pouring water out of the ends of the bells. Keep elbows relaxed and bent. Straighten the wrists, then lower the bells to your sides as you inhale. Don't swing your arms—control those movements.

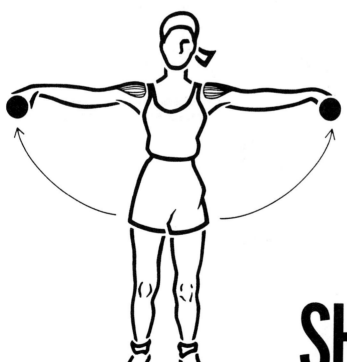

STRAIGHT-ARM RAISES With knees relaxed and feet shoulder width apart, hold weights at your sides. Exhale as you raise dumbbells in an arc until arms extend straight out from the shoulders with wrists slightly bent. Return hands to your sides as you inhale.

SHOULDERS

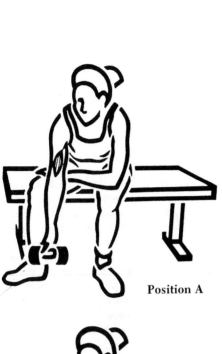

Position A

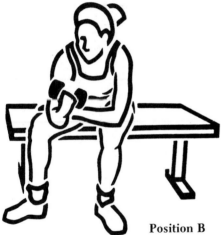

Position B

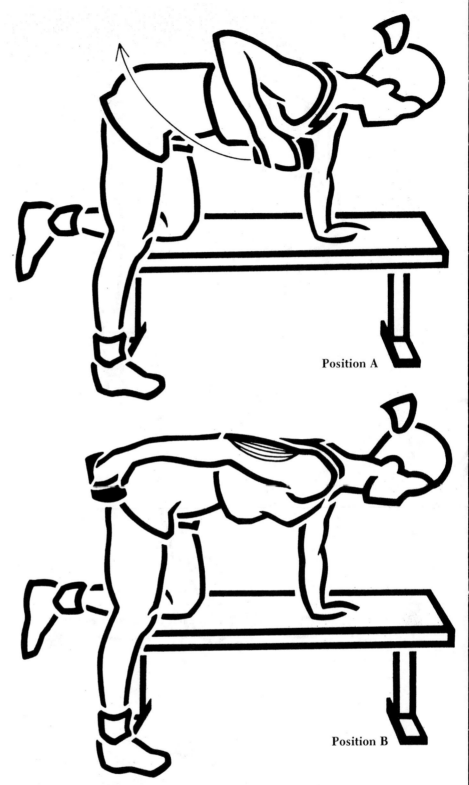

Position A

Position B

CONCENTRATION CURLS Sit on a bench or chair. Leaning forward from the hips with a straight back, place one hand on the opposite knee. With the other hand, grasp a light weight and let your arm hang straight and relaxed. As you exhale, raise the weight by bending your elbow. Be sure that the shoulder doesn't drop and that the effort is felt in the arm, not the shoulder. Inhale as you lower the weight.

ARMS

KICKBACKS Rest your knee and hand on a chair or bench. Keeping the back straight, grasp a light weight in the opposite hand and bring your elbow to waist level so the upper arm is at your side and the forearm hangs straight down. Keeping the upper arm immobile, exhale as you extend the lower arm in a straight line behind you. Bend your elbow to bring the weight to your shoulder and then extend it behind you again. Be sure that your wrist stays straight in line with the lower arm.

Position A   **Position B**

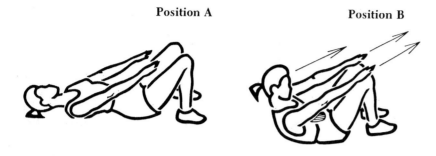

CURL-UPS Lie on your back on a cushioned surface with lower legs at about a 90-degree angle with the floor and feet hip-width apart. Extend arms in front. Raise only your head and shoulders until the upper back is off the floor and your fingertips are on the thighs. Slide your fingers in a path along your thighs to the middle of your kneecaps, then lower your shoulders back to the floor. Exhale as you curl up and inhale as you return to the floor.

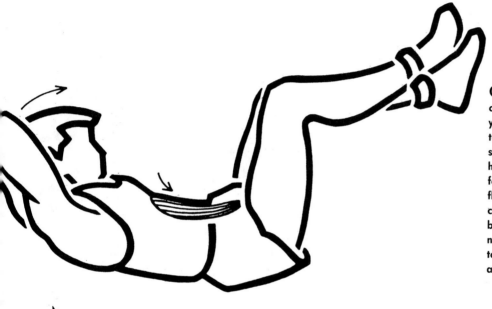

CRUNCHES Lie on your back on a cushioned surface with knees bent. Cross your forearms behind your head (see detail) so that fingertips touch opposite shoulders. This creates a cradle where your head rests. Elevate your legs until they form an L, with thighs perpendicular to the floor and lower legs parallel to it, then cross your ankles. Slowly raise your upper back, using the abdominal muscles, and not straining the neck, then pull your upper torso toward your legs. Exhale as you lift and inhale as you lower.

►**Detail**

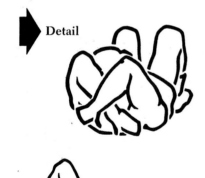

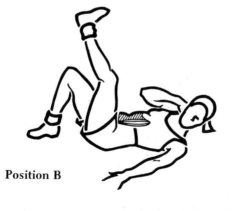

Position B

ONE-LEG LIFT AND TWISTS Lie on your back with one leg bent at the knee and the other leg extended along the mat. The hand on the side of the bent leg is placed behind your head while the arm on the side of the extended leg lies on the mat by your side. Raise the extended leg and your shoulders off the floor touching the bent elbow to the opposite knee. Exhale as you raise and inhale as you lower the foot and the upper body to the mat.

Position A

ABDOMINALS

▶ You have a choice of exercises.
Refer to your strength program chart.

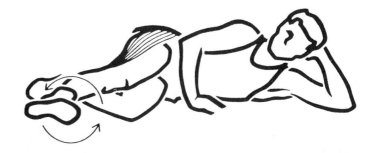

LEG CIRCLES Lie on your side supporting your head with one hand while the other hand rests on the mat in front of your chest for balance. The leg against the floor should bend at the knee, while the upper leg extends out from the body at a 45-degree angle. Keeping your foot flexed so that the toes do *not* point, draw a long circle with your foot. Move in one direction before repeating the movement in the opposite direction.

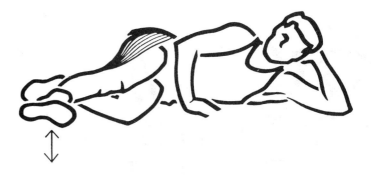

OUTER THIGH LIFTS Lie on your side supporting your head with one hand while the other hand rests on the mat in front of your chest for balance. The leg against the floor should bend at the knee at a 45-degree angle, while the upper leg extends straight out from the body parallel with the thigh of the lower leg. Keeping your foot flexed so that the toes do *not* point, inhale as you lower the extended leg to the floor and exhale as you raise it to hip level.

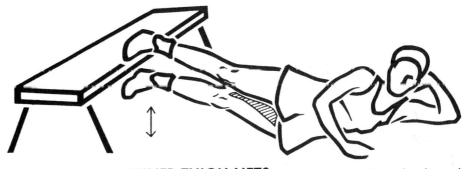

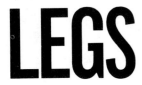

LEGS

INNER THIGH LIFTS Lie on your side with one foot beneath a bench or chair and the upper foot resting on the chair or bench seat. Rest your head on one hand, place the other in front of your chest for balance. Exhale as you lift the lower leg to touch the bottom of the bench; inhale as you lower the leg to the floor. Raise and lower the leg with control.

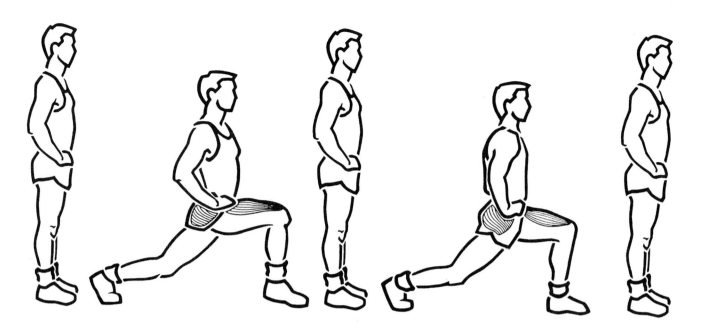

LUNGE WALKS Begin with feet together and hands on hips. You may want to practice the first few sessions with one hand on a wall for balance and control. Keeping your torso erect throughout the exercise, take a giant step forward (two and a half to three feet), and transfer your weight to the forward leg, keeping the heel of the front foot on the ground. The back leg bends slightly and the heel raises, but the knee never touches the ground. Sink until the thigh of the front leg is parallel to the ground. Exhale as you bring the rear leg forward and stand up straight with feet together. Take a giant step forward with the opposite leg, sink, then bring feet together again.

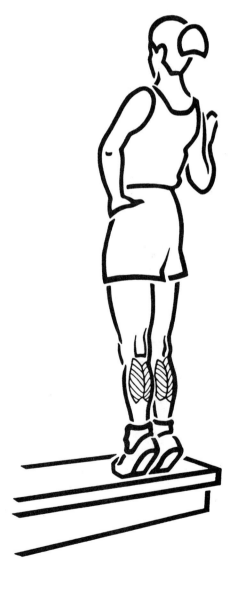

CALF RAISES Stand next to a wall using one hand for balance, with the balls of your feet together on a step or thick telephone book. Keeping knees straight but not locked, inhale as you slowly lower your heels toward the floor and exhale as you rise on the balls of your feet. Be sure that your ankles do not twist outward.

Cool-Down Stretches

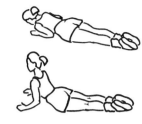

10 Minutes

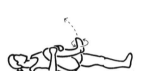 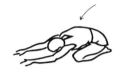
7 THIGH TO CHEST   **13** COBRA

The Cool-Down stretches that end your workout are the same as the stretches that began it—except you'll do them in the opposite order. These illustrations show the correct flow. For instructions on how to perform them turn to pages 44 to 46.

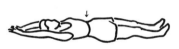
8 FOOT CIRCLES

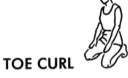
14 SLEEPING CAT
Repeat on the Other Side
Start With Thigh to Chest

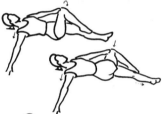
9 BACK TWIST

15 TOE CURL

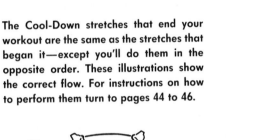
1 SHOULDER ARCH   **4** CHEST PULL

10 KNEE TOUCH

16 VERTICAL RISE

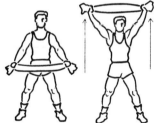
2 SIDE STRETCH

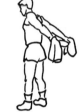 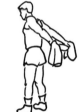 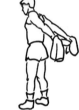
5 THE TORTOISE

11 FULL-BODY STRETCH

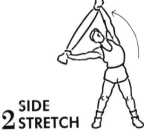
3 ARM PULL

6 KNEE CIRCLES

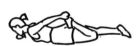
12 THIGH PULL

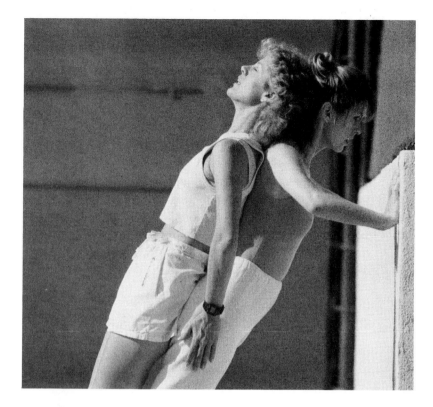

To help a client improve, I'll add more resistance to an exercise by using my body weight.

Little Victories

On a scale of one to ten, how much more fluid and fun is exercise today compared to that first session? If you are scheduling regular sessions and look forward to them—even a little bit—then you are already winning little victories in the battle of the bulge.

After six weeks, you should have trained 18 times. At this point, most of my clients have improved their physical skills and become familiar enough with the program to really start enjoying themselves. I hope you feel the same sense of accomplishment and pleasure in activity.

Once your have those 18 workouts under your shrinking belt, take a few minutes with the tape measure and scale to record your measurements and your weight. You'll find the records in the Appendix. It's now time to move on to *The Train Program* for the next six weeks. Congratulations!

If you skipped more than five workouts and missed out on improvements, don't bother berating yourself. Instead, start training again to make up the sessions you've missed. Staying motivated is most difficult at the beginning of a program. You'll be able to "walk what you talk" by asserting your reasons for wanting an active life-style and "physicalizing" your commitment. Believe in yourself and celebrate little victories all the way!

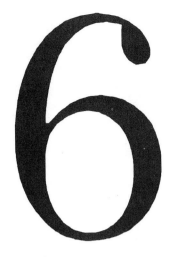

6

If you exercise once a week or less, scored low-to-mid-range on the fitness assessment, and are five to fifteen pounds overweight, then this program is for you.

THE TRAIN PROGRAM

THE
COMPETITIVE OR A HANDLE
EDGE ON HEALTH

5 months and on

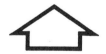

MAINTAIN 10 weeks
(high-end training heart rate)

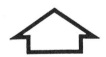

MAINTAIN 4 weeks
(low-end training heart rate)

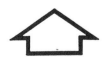

TRAIN
6 weeks

Is your closet a storehouse for dumbbells, ankle weights, maybe even an exercise bike or rowing machine? Some people have no trouble making an exercise resolution. Indeed, they may have made that resolution dozens of times. Unfortunately, after several fervent weeks, all the good intentions seem to end and exercise gets put on hold.

If this scenario sounds familiar, you're ready for *The Train Program*. By following this exercise prescription, you can achieve what you set out to do. The amount of regular exercise you've already been doing has helped set the stage for the weight loss results you will see with this routine. You'll notice improvement in your aerobic capacity because your heart is stronger. You'll even start bolting up stairs. You may feel a distinct relief from back pain as your posture improves. Most important, over the next five months you'll gain self-confidence and realize that your whole life can change because of the physical and psychological benefits of exercise. It will take you five months to move through the Train and Maintain programs, so stay with the order and program requirements as listed to the left.

Training Tips For The Train Program

Make exercise a consistent habit. But don't make it an obsession. It isn't the end of the world if you miss a session—just make sure you complete the next one.

Set specific goals for what you want to accomplish over the next six weeks. While the resolution to exercise is a significant first step, you need to follow through by measuring progress.

If you've started and stopped exercise too many times before, try again, but this time take the workout on the road with you. Take it to the office for lunchtime activity, or to the park with the kids. That way you can leap off the start-and-stop rollercoaster.

Observe how the results of exercise affect your daily life. For example, a real estate agent I train noticed a marked increase in stamina to help her through frantic days of driving, walking, and advising. Are you less winded walking up stairs because you are exercising?

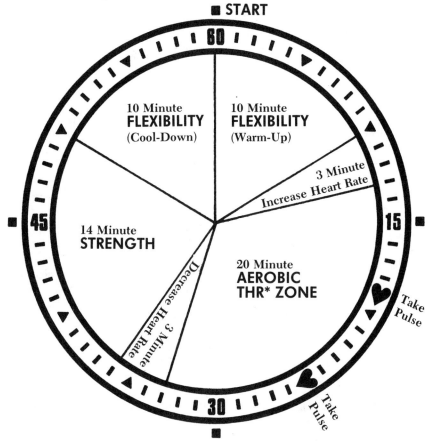

The Train Exercise Hour

1 Hour Workout 3 Times per Week
Optional: 30 Minutes of Aerobic Exercise 1 Day a Week

*Training Heart Rate

Warm-Up Stretches

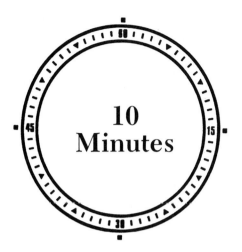

10 Minutes

Equipment

A mat or folded quilt and old bath towel.

Secrets of Stretching

● Warm up your muscles before stretching.
● Exhale as you stretch and inhale as you move into the next position.
● Stretch until you feel tension, then hold the position for 10 to 30 seconds.
● Avoid bouncing.
● Be precise when moving into position.
● Move smoothly and leisurely and *breathe*.
● Perform the stretches in the order listed.

Lower Body

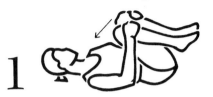

1 THE TORTOISE (for lower back) Lie on your back on the exercise mat and lift knees toward the chest with hands grasping the lower leg beneath the knee. Lengthen your neck and look straight up. Inhale through the nose and exhale through the mouth.
● Transition: Stay in the same position.

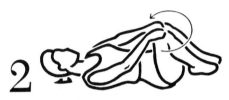

2 KNEE CIRCLES (for lower back) Slide your hands onto kneecaps and circle knees to the right 4 times, keeping abdominals pressed into the lower back so that the base of the spine is against the mat. Gradually make the circles smaller, then reverse the direction for 4 more circles, gradually making the circles larger.
● Transition: Keep one leg toward your chest and extend the other leg straight out along the mat, with the foot flexed so your toes point to the ceiling.

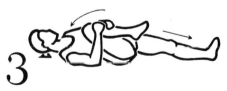

3 THIGH TO CHEST (for lower back) With hands clasped below the knee of the bent leg, exhale as you pull the thigh up and back toward your shoulder. Don't push down toward the ground, but gently pull in an arc toward the shoulder.
● Transition: Keep thigh in the same position, with the other leg still stretched out.

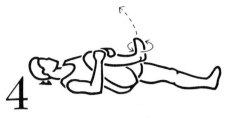

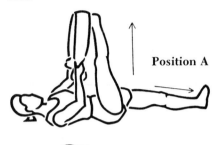

4 FOOT CIRCLES (for ankle) Circle the ankle of the bent leg 4 times to the right, then 4 times to the left.
● Transition: Wrap either a towel or your hands around the ball of the same foot.

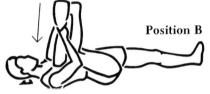

Position A

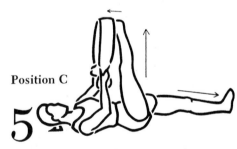

Position B

Position C

5 BOW AND ARROW (for back of leg) Press your heel straight up to the ceiling until the leg is almost straight, but do not lock the knee. Keep your foot flat and the leg extended as you hold the stretch and exhale. Inhale as you bend the knee while using the towel or your hands to help to bring the thigh to your chest, forming a 90-degree angle. The sole of the foot faces the ceiling. Then exhale as you press the heel straight up once more. Throughout these stretches, the leg on the floor is extended.
● Transition: Slowly bring your thigh down to your chest, and put aside the towel. Place the foot of this leg on the knee of your outstretched leg.

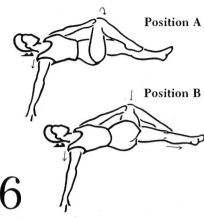

Position A

Position B

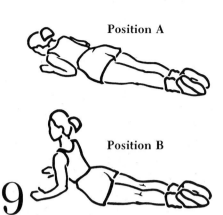

Position A

Position B

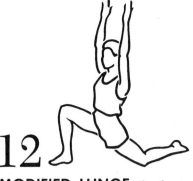

12

MODIFIED LUNGE (for front of leg) Using the muscles in your thighs, move one foot forward until the knee is perpendicular to the floor and in line with the heel. Move the pelvis forward to stretch the back leg. The back thigh should form a 45-degree angle with the floor, and the top of the foot should be flat against the mat. Adjust your front foot to keep the knee over the toe. Raise your hands over your head, keeping the torso erect as you exhale. If you need to stabilize your balance place both hands on the front knee.

● **Transition:** Inhale as your pelvis moves backward to straighten your forward leg, and place your hands either on your knee or on the mat for balance.

6

BACK TWIST (for back) Grasp the outside of the bent knee with the opposite hand. Stretch the other hand away from the body, level with the shoulder. Gently push the bent leg toward the floor while keeping your shoulders square on the mat. Exhale as you gently press downward, and inhale as you hold the stretch for at least 30 seconds. Use 3 or more exhalations to relax the leg toward the floor. Finally, turn the head away from the direction of the twist.

● **Transition:** Release the stretch and straighten your head.

9

COBRA (for back and abdominals) Pressing the palms of the hands into the floor lift the upper body without collapsing the shoulders, using the bent forearms to raise the torso while pelvis remains on the floor.

● **Transition:** Lower your torso until you are flat on the mat. Push yourself up until you are sitting on knees and feet.

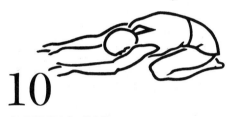

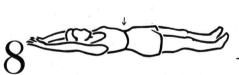

7

KNEE TOUCH (for back) With both hands, grasp beneath the knee. Lift your head, neck, and upper back from the floor and touch your kneecap with your nose.

● **Transition:** Return your head, upper body, and bent leg to the mat.

10

SLEEPING CAT (for lower back) Exhale as you bend from the waist and extend your arms out in front of you until your chest is on your thighs.

● **Transition:** Raise your torso and rest on hands and knees.

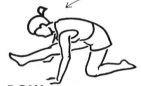

13

FORWARD BOW (for back of leg) Bending from the waist, exhale as you lower your chest toward your thigh. Be sure you are not sitting back, but that your stabilizing knee is directly under the hip, and your buttocks are over the knee.

● **Transition:** Bend the stretching leg so you are on your knees and start the *Modified Lunge* and *Forward Bow* on the other side.

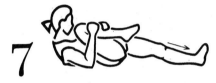

8

FULL-BODY STRETCH (for all major muscles) Stretch your arms overhead and extend both legs as you exhale. Press abdominals toward the floor to keep lower back flat.

● **First Transition:** Start the series with *Thigh to Chest* on the other side.

● **Second Transition:** After completing the series on the opposite side through the *Full-Body Stretch*, roll onto your stomach, bringing hands under the shoulders with forearms flat on the floor, and head looking down at the mat.

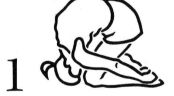

11

RABBIT (for upper back and top of shoulders) Place the crown of your head, the baby's "soft spot," onto the floor as close to your knees as possible. Firmly wrap the palms of your hands around the soles of your arches. Deeply inhale, then exhale as you slowly lift the buttocks into the air while the arms straighten. You will feel this stretch in the upper shoulders.

● **Transition:** Roll upright until your torso is erect and hands are next to your knees.

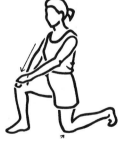

14

VERTICAL RISE (to protect back upon standing) Bring the front foot back so that your thigh parallels the floor. Place both hands on top of the knee in front of you, and pull the toes of your rear foot forward. Press down on the knee, stabilizing your balance as you stand up.

Warm-Up Stretches Continue

Warm-Up Stretches

Upper Body

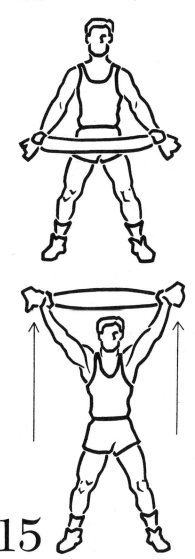

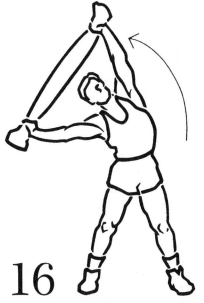

16

SIDE STRETCH (for sides of the trunk) Keeping the towel taut, exhale as you use one hand to pull the towel downward, bending the trunk to one side. Prevent your back from arching by tightening the abdominal muscles. Increase the stretch for 3 deep breaths by pulling down on the towel with the lower arm, continuing to bend to the side. Slowly stand straight and repeat the stretch on the opposite side.

● Transition: Stand erect, knees slightly bent, towel over head. Bend your elbows, lowering the stretched-out towel behind your head.

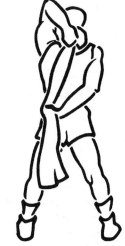

18

ARM PULL (for back of arm) Bring your free arm behind your back to grab the towel at a comfortable distance. The arm holding the towel should be near the ear with the elbow pointing forward. Pull down on the towel to stretch the back of the bent arm as you exhale. Hold the stretch for 3 deep breaths, keeping the tension in the towel constant. Then switch the towel to the other hand and repeat the stretch.

● Transition: Let go of the towel with the upper arm and extend both arms downward with palms facing toward the rear. Grasp both ends and stretch the towel behind your back.

15

SHOULDER ARCH (for shoulders) Taking the towel in both hands, stand with your feet farther than shoulder-width apart with arms straight. Without locking your elbows, raise both your arms in an arc, keeping the towel taut, until hands swing behind the head. Lower your hands to the thighs and repeat the movement smoothly 5 times.

● Transition: Hold the last stretch above the head and bend the knees slightly.

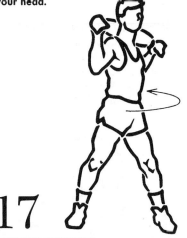

17

WAIST TWISTS (for back and trunk) With toes and hips pointing straight ahead and abdominals tightened, anchor your hips by pressing the abdominal muscles toward the back. Twist your trunk slowly in one direction as far as you can without letting the hips turn. Hold the towel in a straight line to keep your elbows back, and face forward. Twist to the opposite side, then alternate sides 8 times.

● Transition: Bend your elbow so the towel is hanging to the floor behind you.

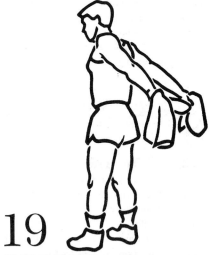

19

CHEST PULL (for chest) Holding the towel in a straight line, lift both arms straight up until you feel the stretch in the chest and shoulder muscles. Take 3 deep breaths in this position while the muscles relax.

Aerobic Conditioning

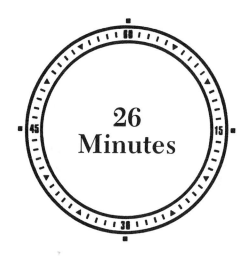

Activity Swim, walk, stationary cycle, rowing machine, low-impact dance exercise, or a combination of these activities.

Intensity 3 minutes to elevate heart rate—20 minutes in your personal heart rate zone—3 minutes to decrease heart rate to 100–110 beats per minute

The Train Heart Rate Chart

Age	Resting Heart Rate	Train 55–75% (RPE Scale) 10–14
beats per minute—10-second count		
Round Up to Nearest Age and Resting Heart Rate		
20 years	60	137–165 **23–28**
	70	142–168 **24–28**
	80	146–170 **24–28**
30 years	60	132–158 **23–26**
	70	136–160 **23–27**
	80	140–162 **23–27**
40 years	60	126–150 **21–25**
	70	131–153 **22–26**
	80	135–155 **23–26**
50 years	60	121–143 **20–24**
	70	125–145 **21–24**
	80	130–148 **22–25**
60+ years	60	115–135 **19–23**
	70	120–138 **20–23**
	80	124–140 **21–23**

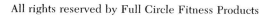

Aerobic Training Tips

● Monitor your exercise intensity twice during each aerobic workout: Take your pulse at 8 minutes and 15 minutes into the activity.
● Take the time to learn the proper form and method for each activity.
● Move continuously for at least 20 minutes.
● If you exercise outdoors, accommodate to the weather.

Strength Training

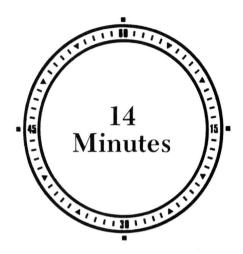

14 Minutes

Equipment

- 3–5-pound dumbbells for women
- 5–8-pound dumbbells for men
- "Record Your Workout" chart

Strength Training Secrets

- It is important to understand the execution of each exercise.
- Close your eyes, concentrate, and use your "mind's eye" to focus on, or isolate, the muscles you are using.
- Exhale on the contraction—the lift or push—and inhale during the opposite movement.
- Use slow, fully controlled movements in both directions without permitting momentum to do any of the work.
- Move through the complete range of motion that you can achieve.
- Sets are a defined number of repetitions (reps) done consecutively (i.e., 1–2 sets, or times)
- Use the suggested resistance or weight for each program.
- Keep exercises in the indicated sequence.

The Train Program

CHEST
1. Incline Push-ups, 12 reps × 1 set
or
1. Modified Push-ups, 12 reps × 1 set

BACK
1. One-Arm Rows, dumbbells, 12 reps × 1 set

SHOULDERS
1. Military Presses, dumbbells, 12 reps × 1 set
2. Upright Rows, dumbbells, 12 reps × 1 set

ARMS
1. Alternate Curls, dumbbells, 12 reps × 1 set
2. Dips, 12 reps × 1 set

ABDOMINALS
1. Curl-ups, 16 reps × 1 set
2. Crunches, 16 reps × 1 set
3. Side Crunches, 12 reps (each side) × 1 set
4. Bicycles, 12 reps (each side) × 1 set

LEGS
1. Leg Circles, 12 forward and 12 backward (each leg)
2. Outer Thigh Lifts, 32 reps × 1 set (each leg)
3. Inner Thigh Lifts, 32 reps × 1 set (each leg)
or
1. Lunge Walks, 24 reps × 1 set
2. Calf Raises, 24 reps × 1 set

You have a choice of exercises.
Refer to your strength program chart.

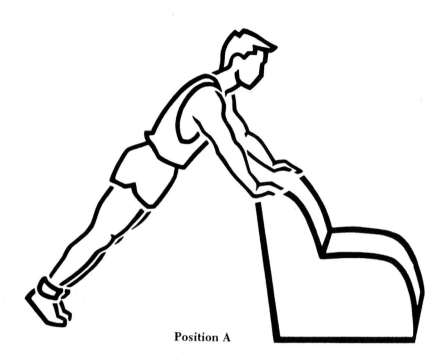

Position A

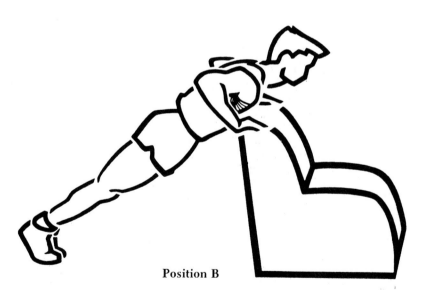

Position B

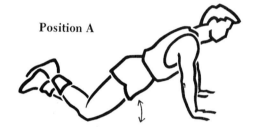

Position A

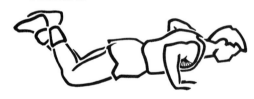

Position B

MODIFIED PUSH-UPS Resting on your hands and knees, position hands shoulder-width apart with fingers pointing forward, and feet lifted and crossed at the ankles. Lean forward and lower your entire body slowly as you inhale, touch the floor, then lift to the starting position while exhaling. Keep abdominal muscles contracted and back and hips in a straight line at all times.

INCLINE PUSH-UPS Stand an arm's length away from a low bench, couch, or other sturdy surface with hands shoulder-width apart. Take one or two steps farther back. Keep your body straight in one line from the top of your head to your heels, with heels raised. Support your back by contracting the abdominal muscles. As your elbows go out to the side, lower your chest to the bench while you inhale. Then exhale as you press your body away.

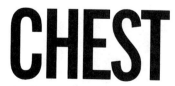

CHEST

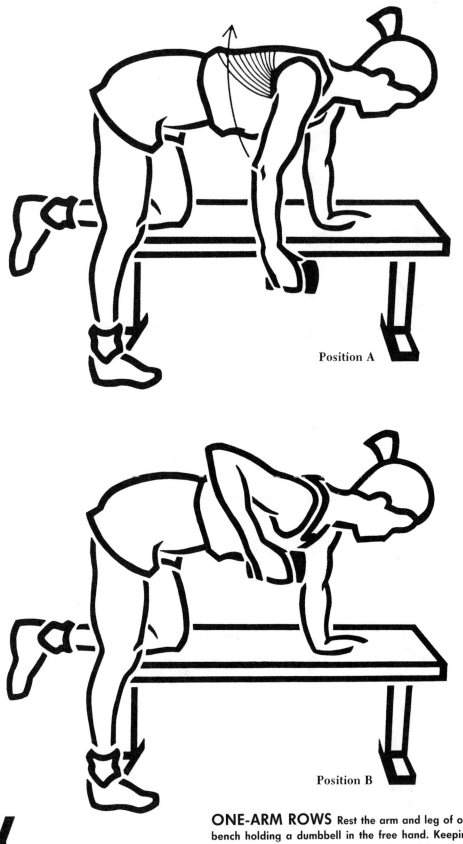

Position A

Position B

BACK

ONE-ARM ROWS Rest the arm and leg of one side on a low bench holding a dumbbell in the free hand. Keeping your shoulder immobile and your back flat, raise the weight straight up along the side of your body to just below the armpit. Exhale as you lift the bell, inhale as you lower it.

Position A

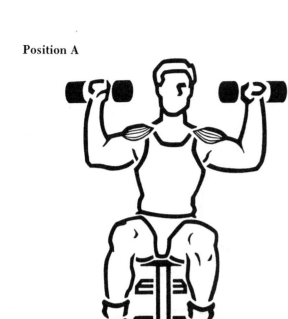

Position B

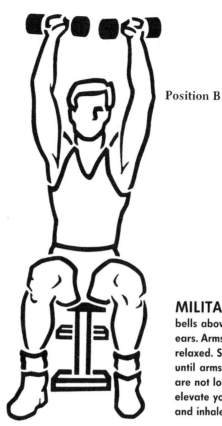

MILITARY PRESSES Hold dumb-bells above your shoulders, level with the ears. Arms will be L-shaped with shoulders relaxed. Slowly raise the bells straight up until arms are fully extended, but elbows are not locked. Do not arch your back or elevate your shoulders. Exhale as you lift and inhale as you lower the weights.

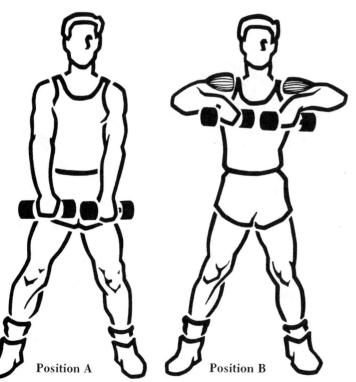

Position A   Position B

UPRIGHT ROWS Stand with your feet slightly farther than shoulder-width apart, knee slightly bent. Hold weights in front of thighs and lean forward slightly to avoid arching your back when you lift. With shoulders relaxed, bend your elbows to lift the dumbbells straight up to your collarbone. Exhale as you lift and inhale as you lower the bells.

SHOULDERS

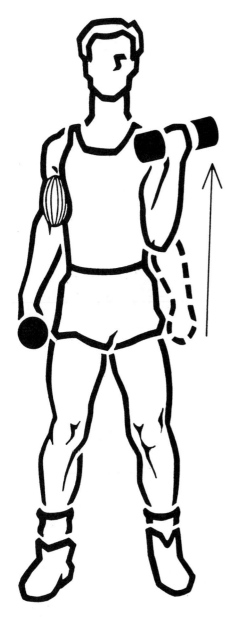

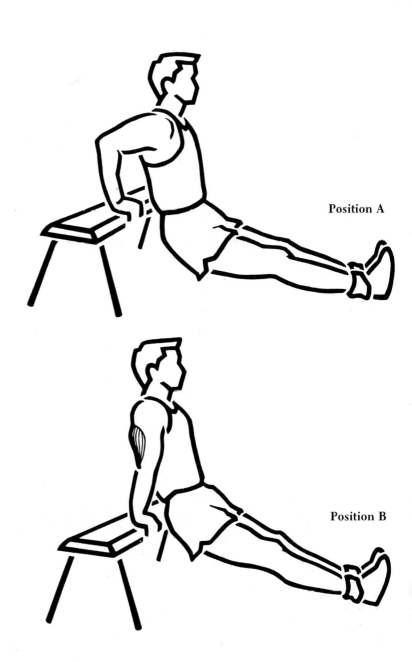

Position A

Position B

ALTERNATE CURLS Stand with your feet slightly farther than shoulder-width apart and knees slightly bent. Hold weights at your sides and lean forward slightly to avoid arching your back when you lift. Keeping shoulders down and elbows at your side, raise the forearm only to lift the weight to the shoulder. Lift one dumbbell at a time, alternating sides.

ARMS

DIPS Sit on the edge of a sturdy chair or bench, with legs together and hands resting on the seat next to your buttocks. Support your upper body with your hands and step forward, one foot at a time, so that both legs are extended fully and your weight is balanced on your heels. Keeping your back straight and shoulders down, slowly lower your body until the upper arm is parallel to the floor and elbows point straight behind you. Keep the body close to the bench. Inhale as you lower and exhale as you push back up.

Position A

Position B

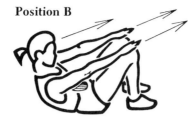

CURL-UPS Lie on your back on a cushioned surface with lower legs at about a 90-degree angle with the floor and feet hip-width apart. Extend arms in front. Raise only your head and shoulders until the upper back is off the floor and your fingertips are on the thighs. Slide your fingers in a path along your thighs to the middle of your kneecap, then lower your shoulders back to the floor. Exhale as you curl up and inhale as you return to the floor.

Detail

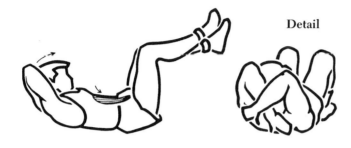

CRUNCHES Lie on your back on a cushioned surface with knees bent. Cross your forearms behind your head so that fingertips touch opposite shoulders. This creates a cradle where your head rests. Elevate your legs until they form an L, with thighs perpendicular to the floor and lower legs parallel to it, then cross your ankles. Slowly raise your upper back, using the abdominal muscles, and not straining the neck, then pull your upper torso toward your legs. Exhale as you lift and inhale as you lower.

SIDE CRUNCHES Lie on your back with knees bent. Cross legs at the knee, then let them fall gently, in one unit, to one side. Lift your head and shoulders with arms reaching in the opposite direction from your legs. Roll up with straight arms, slowly exhaling as you reach diagonally. Do not roll all the way down.

BICYCLES Lie on your back on a cushioned surface with hands behind head. Lift both legs into an L shape, keeping the lower leg parallel to the floor. Raise your shoulders from the mat and alternately touch an elbow to the opposite knee while moving your thighs slightly back and forth. Keep your lower back pressed into the mat and contract your abdominal muscles to support the action. Touching the elbow to both sides is 1 repetition.

ABDOMINALS

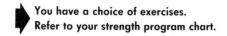 You have a choice of exercises.
Refer to your strength program chart.

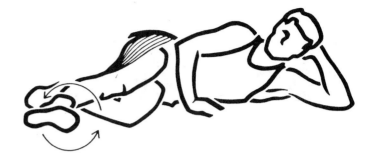

LEG CIRCLES Lie on your side supporting your head with one hand while the other hand rests on the mat in front of your chest for balance. The leg against the floor should bend at the knee, while the upper leg extends out from the body at a 45-degree angle. Keeping your foot flexed so that the toes do *not* point, draw a long circle with your foot. Move in one direction before repeating the movement in the opposite direction.

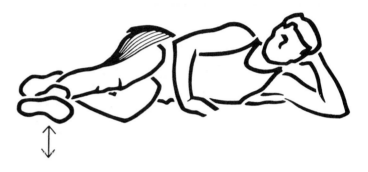

OUTER THIGH LIFTS Lie on your side supporting your head with one hand while the other hand rests on the mat in front of your chest for balance. The leg against the floor should bend at the knee at a 45-degree angle, while the upper leg extends straight out from the body parallel with the thigh of the lower leg. Keeping your foot flexed so that the toes do *not* point, inhale as you lower the extended leg to the floor and exhale as you raise it to hip level.

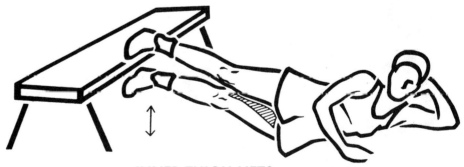

LEGS

INNER THIGH LIFTS Lie on your side with one foot beneath a bench or chair and the upper foot resting on the chair or bench seat. Rest your head on one hand, place the other in front of your chest for balance. Exhale as you lift the lower leg to touch the bottom of the bench; inhale as you lower the leg to the floor. Raise and lower the leg with control.

70   THE TRAIN PROGRAM

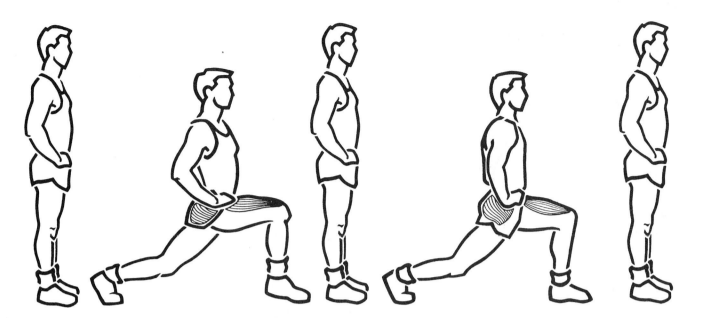

LUNGE WALKS Begin with feet together and hands on hips. You may want to practice the first few sessions with one hand on a wall for balance and control. Keeping your torso erect throughout the exercise, take a giant step forward (two and a half to three feet), and transfer your weight to the forward leg, keeping the heel of the front foot on the ground. The back leg bends slightly and the heel raises, but the knee never touches the ground. Sink until the thigh of the front leg is parallel to the ground. Exhale as you bring the rear leg forward and stand up straight with feet together. Take a giant step forward with the opposite leg, sink, then bring feet together again.

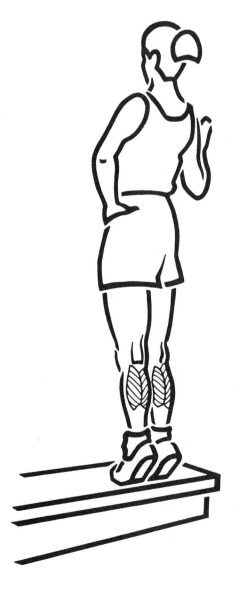

CALF RAISES Stand next to a wall using one hand for balance, with the balls of your feet together on a step or thick telephone book. Keeping knees straight but not locked, inhale as you slowly lower your heels toward the floor and exhale as you rise on the balls of your feet. Be sure that your ankles do not twist outward.

Cool-Down Stretches

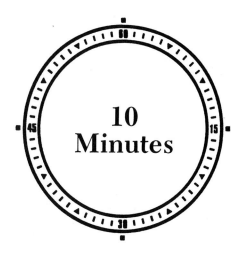

10 Minutes

The Cool-Down stretches that end your workout are almost the same as the stretches that began it—except you'll do them in the opposite order. These illustrations show the correct flow. For instructions on how to perform them, turn to pages 60 to 62.

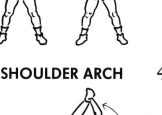 **7 THIGH TO CHEST**

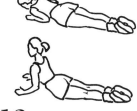 **13 COBRA**

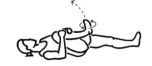 **8 FOOT CIRCLES**

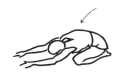 **14 SLEEPING CAT**

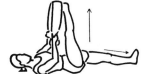 **9 BOW AND ARROW**

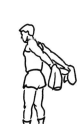 **15 RABBIT**

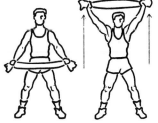 **1 SHOULDER ARCH**   **4 CHEST PULL**

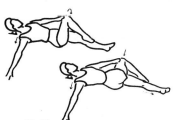 **10 BACK TWIST**

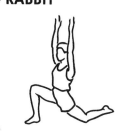 **16 MODIFIED LUNGE**

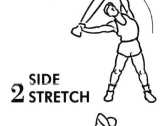 **2 SIDE STRETCH**   **5 THE TORTOISE**

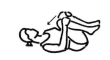

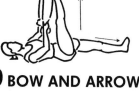 **11 KNEE TOUCH**

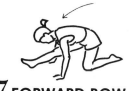 **17 FORWARD BOW**

▶ Repeat on the Other Side
Start With Modified Lunge

3 ARM PULL   **6 KNEE CIRCLES**

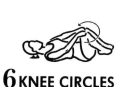

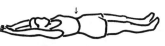 **12 FULL-BODY STRETCH**

▶ Repeat on the Other Side
Start With Thigh to Chest

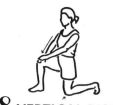 **18 VERTICAL RISE**

"Physicalizing"

You probably have a whole new definition of "getting physical" if you have followed *The Train Program* for one hour 18 to 24 times during the past six weeks. Fast walking and stretching muscles after work is much more fun than relying on taking out the garbage for exercise.

This is a good time to measure your progress by repeating the fitness assessments located in the Appendix. Record your results on the personal fitness progress chart and note your weight and measurements just for the sake of comparison at a later date. If you have kept exercising, strong and steady, you will be in the average range for push-ups. If you started with the *Gain* routine you're not doing wall push-ups at all. Flexibility will be better and so will the number of sit-ups you can do. This is when most of my clients start *feeling* their bodies and hear comments about their visual difference. Take a look at yourself; it *is* worth the effort!

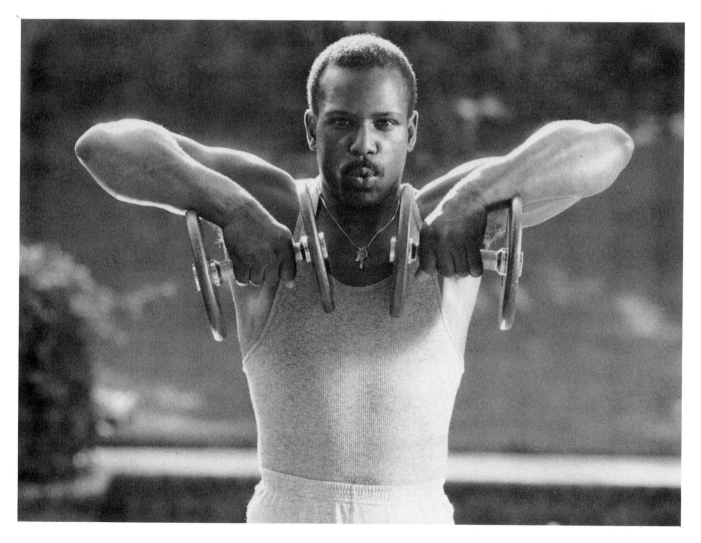

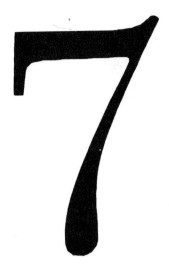

7

The Maintain Program is the place to be if you already exercise two or more times per week and scored at mid- to upper-range on the fitness assessments.

THE MAINTAIN PROGRAM

Maybe you meet your best friend every Saturday for a game of tennis and a run around the high school's track. Perhaps you yawn out of bed and tumble onto the floor for a few sit-ups, then walk around the business park on your lunch hour twice a week. Despite this effort, do you feel you are not making any progress?

You're already doing well because you have some exercise in your life, but by structuring and planning activity you can make tangible gains. *The Maintain Program* is unique in that there are two stages of conditioning within it that provide direction and an opportunity for measurable progress. It can help you lose that last five pounds or permanently toss away the cigarettes. The intensity prescriptions in the Maintain routine increase stamina, plus provide a different warm-up and cool-down stretch routine to keep the challenge. It will take four months to move a moderate exerciser through *The Maintain Program,* so stay with the requirements as listed below.

Your initial capacity for exercise affects the prescription of this stage in physical fitness. When you are graduating from the Train routine into the Maintain routine stay with the time and intensity requirement from your original program. For *The Gain Program,* see page 42. For *The Train Program,* see page 58.

Training Tips For The Maintain Program

Record your measurements at 6 and 12 weeks. Now you can see the positive impact of exercise and gain motivation.

Begin alternating among aerobic modes. Bicycle one day and run during the next session. Use a friend's rowing machine every few weeks. It's fairly easy to change aerobic modes and it helps keep exercise interesting by adding variety.

If you have difficulty exercising in your training heart rate zone begin with a walk. If you can't maintain the full

**THE
COMPETITIVE** OR **A HANDLE
EDGE** **ON HEALTH**

4 months and on

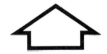

MAINTAIN 10 weeks
(high-end training heart rate)

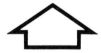

MAINTAIN 6 weeks
(low-end training heart rate)

25 minutes of aerobic exercise in each session, start or finish with walking and slowly increase the time you cycle, jog, or row at your appropriate intensity.

Change the sequence of the weight training exercises. One session work from the top of your body to the bottom, on the next exercise day work from bottom to top. Do not change the order of the exercises though, because you risk not working the muscle groups systematically.

Schedule exercise into your week. And keep those appointments because only your consistent effort will bring improvement.

Because you have a base level of physical conditioning, there are more exercises in each hour. Keep a clock nearby to keep yourself on schedule so that you stay within your hourly commitment.

Don't leave home without your program. Vacation where you can bicycle or run. Meet a friend for a fun hike instead of a drink.

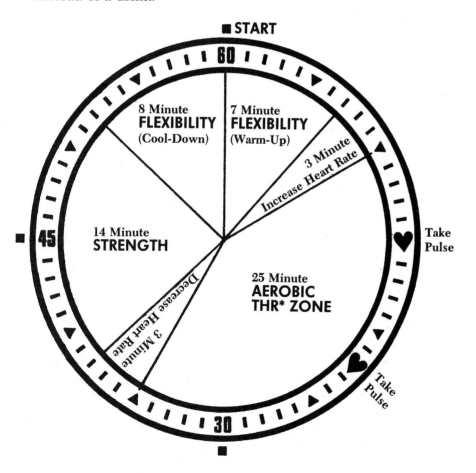

The Maintain Exercise Hour
**1 Hour Workout 3 Times per Week and
30 Minutes of Aerobic Exercise 1 Day a Week**

*Training Heart Rate

Warm-Up Stretches

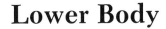

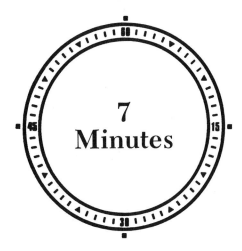

7 Minutes

Equipment

A mat or folded quilt and old bath towel.

Secrets of Stretching

● Warm up your muscles before stretching.
● Exhale as you stretch and inhale as you move into the next position.
● Stretch until you feel tension, then hold the position for 10 to 30 seconds.
● Avoid bouncing.
● Be precise when moving into position.
● Move smoothly and leisurely and breathe.
● Perform the stretches in the order listed.

Lower Body

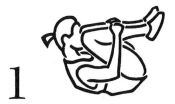

1

THE EGG (for abdominals) Lie on your back on a cushioned surface and bring both legs toward your chest. Press the abdominals toward your back and exhale as you grasp your shins and gently pull your legs to your chest while lifting your head between your knees.
● Transition: Return your head to the floor and extend one leg with the foot flexed so toes point to the ceiling.

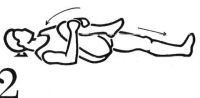

2

THIGH TO CHEST (for lower back) With hands clasped below the knee of the bent leg, exhale as you pull the thigh up and back toward your shoulder. Don't push down toward the ground, but gently pull in an arc toward the shoulder.
● Transition: Place arms and legs on the mat.

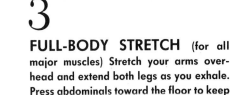

3

FULL-BODY STRETCH (for all major muscles) Stretch your arms overhead and extend both legs as you exhale. Press abdominals toward the floor to keep lower back flat.
● Transition: Bring your arms to the side of your hips with palms facing up.

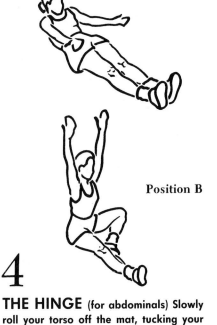

Position A

Position B

4

THE HINGE (for abdominals) Slowly roll your torso off the mat, tucking your chin to your chest and reaching forward. Raise your arms overhead and exhale as you lift yourself up.
● Transition: Keeping arms elevated, bend one leg and place the sole of the foot next to the knee of the extended leg. If the backs of your legs are tight, use a towel.

Position A

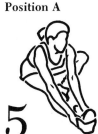 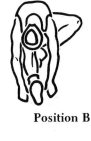

Position B

5

SINGLE LEG PULL (for back of leg) Bend forward from the hips, placing either your hands or a towel around the arch of the extended foot. Keep your back as straight as possible and bend the elbows as you exhale to increase the stretch. Put aside the towel and exhale as you lower the chest to the thigh. Throughout the stretch your foot points to the ceiling and hands slide alongside the extended leg.
● Transition: Raise your torso and bend the extended leg so you sit cross-legged.

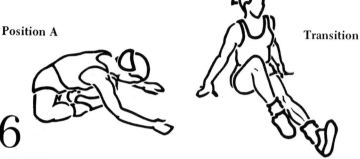

Position A

Transition

6

WIGWAM (for buttocks and lower back) Turn toward the inside leg and lower your upper body to the thigh. Arms are outstretched on either side of the knee.

● Transition: Roll up until you are sitting erect and facing forward. Place your hands behind you for support bringing the outside foot flat on the floor. Extend the inside leg with toes flexed to point toward the ceiling.

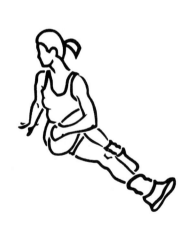

7

SEATED BACK TWIST (for entire back) Place the foot of the leg you have been working on the outside of the knee of the extended leg. Twist your torso toward the bent leg, placing your elbow on the outside of the bent knee. Balance your body with the fingertips of the hand behind you, exhaling as you pull that shoulder into a straight line with the forward shoulder. Be sure the hip of the side you are working is placed on the mat.

● Transition: Face forward and bring the soles of both feet together.

8

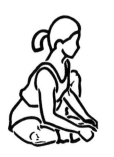

DOUBLE LEG PULL (for inner thigh) Taking hold of the toes of the feet bring the elbows inside of the knees. Exhale as you bend the elbows pulling the upper body, with a flat back, toward the feet.

● Transition: Release your feet and roll slowly down to the floor and onto your back. Place the foot of the bent-knee leg on the floor and rest the foot of the stretching leg on the knee.

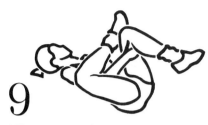

9

HIP STRETCH (for buttocks) Place your hands beneath the knee of the leg on the floor and exhale as you bend the elbows to pull the leg toward the shoulder. Keep the other leg relaxed and at a 90-degree angle to the knee.

● First Transition: Start series with *Thigh to Chest* on the other side.
● Second Transition: After completing the series on the opposite side through the *Hip Stretch*, roll onto your side.

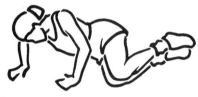

10

HORIZONTAL RISE (to protect back upon rising) Use your arms to walk the upper body into an upright position.

● Transition: Shift your weight to your knees.

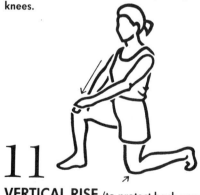

11

VERTICAL RISE (to protect back upon standing) Bring one foot forward so that your thigh parallels the floor. Place both hands on top of the knee in front of you, and pull the toes of your rear foot forward. Press down on the knee, stabilizing your balance as you stand up.

Warm-Up Stretches Continue

Warm-Up Stretches

Upper Body

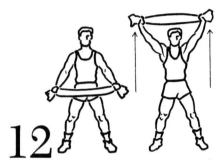

12

SHOULDER ARCH (for shoulders) Taking the towel in both hands, stand with your feet farther than shoulder-width apart with arms straight. Without locking your elbows, raise both your arms in an arc, keeping the towel taut, until hands swing behind the head. Lower your hands to the thighs and repeat the movement smoothly 5 times.

● Transition: Hold the last stretch above the head and bend the knees slightly.

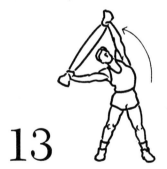

13

SIDE STRETCH (for sides of the trunk) Keeping the towel taut, exhale as you use one hand to pull the towel downward, bending the trunk to one side. Prevent your back from arching by tightening the abdominal muscles. Increase the stretch for 3 deep breaths by pulling down on the towel with the lower arm, continuing to bend to the side. Slowly stand straight and repeat the stretch on the opposite side.

● Transition: Stand erect, knees slightly bent, towel over head. Bend your elbows, lowering the stretched-out towel behind your head.

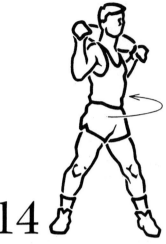

14

WAIST TWISTS (for back and trunk) With toes and hips pointing straight ahead and abdominals tightened, anchor your hips by pressing the abdominal muscles toward the back. Twist your trunk slowly in one direction as far as you can without letting the hips turn. Hold the towel in a straight line to keep your elbows back, and face forward. Twist to the opposite side, then alternate sides 8 times.

● Transition: Face forward and release your grip from one end of the towel.

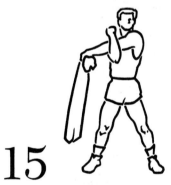

15

SHOULDER PULL (for shoulder) Extend the hand holding the towel straight in front of you. Your free hand, palm up, travels under the extended arm and hooks around the upper arm just above the elbow. Use the hooked arm to pull the straight arm toward the middle of your body. Hold for 3 breaths, then transfer the towel to the other hand and repeat the stretch on that side.

● Transition: Bring the hand holding the towel over your head, then bend your elbow so the towel is hanging to the floor behind you.

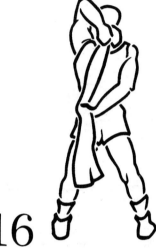

16

ARM PULL (for back of arm) Bring your free arm behind your back to grab the towel at a comfortable distance. The arm holding the towel should be near the ear with the elbow pointing forward. Pull down on the towel to stretch the back of the bent arm as you exhale. Hold the stretch for 3 deep breaths, keeping the tension in the towel constant. Then switch the towel to the other hand and repeat the stretch.

● Transition: Let go of the towel with the upper arm and extend both arms downward with palms facing toward the rear. Grasp both ends and stretch the towel behind your back.

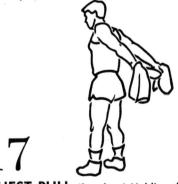

17

CHEST PULL (for chest) Holding the towel in a straight line, lift both arms straight up until you feel the stretch in the chest and shoulder muscles. Take 3 deep breaths in this position while the muscles relax.

Aerobic Conditioning

Activity Swim, walk, cycle, rowing machine, dance exercise, cross-country ski machine, jog, run, or a combination of these.

Intensity 3 minutes to elevate heart rate—25 minutes in your personal heart rate zone—3 minutes to decrease heart rate to 100–110 beats per minute

The Maintain Heart Rate Chart

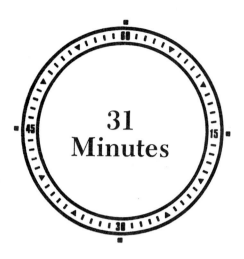

		(RPE Scale) 11–15
Round Up to Nearest Age and Resting Heart Rate beats per minute—10-second count		
Age	Resting Heart Rate	Maintain 60–80%
20 years	60	144–172 **24–29**
	70	148–174 **25–29**
	80	152–176 **25–29**
30 years	60	138–164 **23–27**
	70	142–166 **24–28**
	80	146–168 **24–28**
40 years	60	132–156 **22–26**
	70	136–158 **23–26**
	80	140–160 **23–27**
50 years	60	126–148 **21–25**
	70	130–150 **22–25**
	80	134–152 **22–25**
60+ years	60	120–140 **20–23**
	70	124–142 **21–24**
	80	128–144 **21–24**

Aerobic Training Tips

- Monitor your exercise intensity twice during each aerobic workout: Take your pulse at 8 minutes and 15 minutes into the activity.
- Take the time to learn the proper form and method for each activity.
- Move continuously for at least 20 minutes.
- If you exercise outdoors, accommodate to the weather.

Strength Training

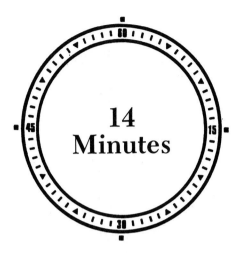

14 Minutes

Equipment

- 5- to 10-pound dumbbells for women
- 8- to 12-pound dumbbells for men
- flat exercise bench
- "Record Your Workout" chart

Strength Training Secrets

- Pay attention to the execution of each exercise.
- Concentrate on the muscles you are using.
- Exhale on the contraction—the lift or push—and inhale during the opposite movement.
- Use slow, fully controlled movements in both directions without permitting momentum to do any of the work.
- Move through the complete range of motion that you can achieve.
- Sets are a defined number of repetitions done consecutively (i.e., 1–2 sets, or times).
- Keep exercises in the indicated sequence.
- Work up to 15 repetitions, then increase the weight of dumbbells by 2–3 pounds every 4 weeks.

The Maintain Program

CHEST
1. **Modified Push-ups**, 16 reps × 1 set
2. **Flyes**, dumbbells, 12 reps × 1 set

BACK
1. **Double Rows**, dumbbells, 12 reps × 1 set

SHOULDERS
1. **Military Presses**, dumbbells, 12 reps × 1 set
2. **Upright Rows**, dumbbells, 12 reps × 1 set

ARMS
1. **Alternate Curls**, dumbbells, 12 reps × 1 set
2. **French Curls**, dumbbells, 12 reps × 1 set

ABDOMINALS
Crunches, 24 reps × 1 set
Curl-ups, 24 reps × 1 set
Bicycles, 24 reps (each leg) × 1 set
Pops, 16 reps × 1 set

LEGS
1. **Knee-ups**, 32 reps × 1 set (each leg)
2. **Outer Thigh Lifts**, 32 reps × 1 set (each leg)
3. **Corkscrews**, 32 reps × 1 set (each leg)
4. **Inner Thigh Lifts**, 32 reps × 1 set (each leg)
or
1. **Lunge Walks**, 16 reps × 2 sets
2. **Calf Raises**, 24 reps × 2 sets

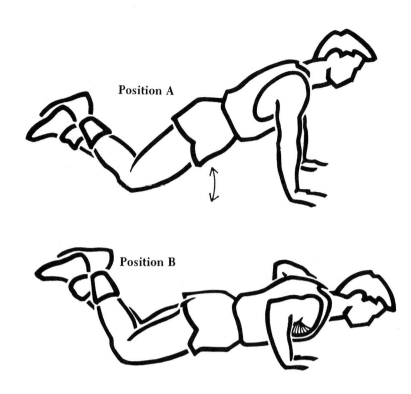

Position A

Position B

MODIFIED PUSH-UPS Resting on your hands and knees, position hands shoulder-width apart with fingers pointing forward, and feet lifted and crossed at the ankles. Lean forward and lower your entire body slowly as you inhale, touch the floor, then lift to the starting position while exhaling. Keep abdominal muscles contracted and back and hips in a straight line at all times.

FLYES Lie on an exercise bench with knees bent and feet on the bench to keep your back flat. Hold dumbbells over your chest with hands together, keeping your elbows slightly bent. As you inhale, lower the bells in a circular arc until they are level with your chest. Your elbows should be pointing to the floor but not lower than your wrists. Exhale as you raise the dumbbells to bring them together over your chest.

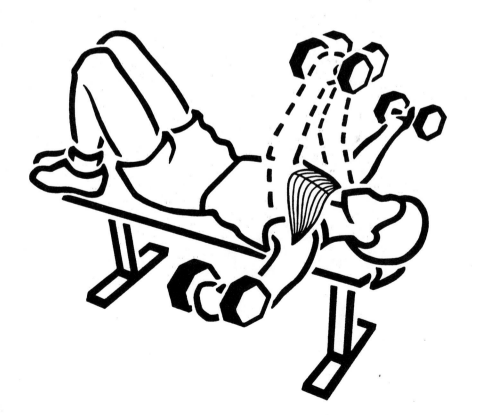

CHEST

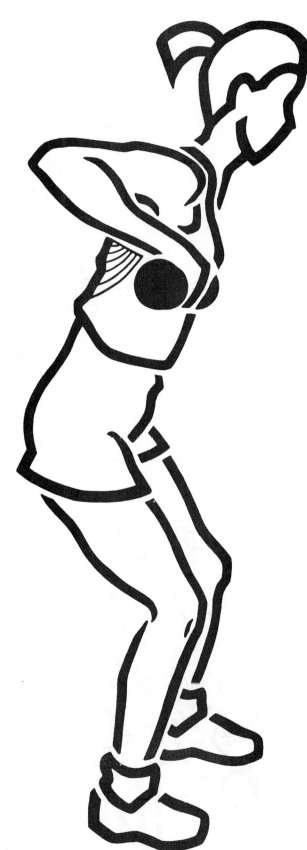

DOUBLE ROWS Bend forward slightly from the waist with knees bent and feet shoulder-width apart. With a weight in each hand, let your arms hang relaxed at your sides, palms facing to the rear. Keep your back straight as you raise the weights to your armpits *without* lifting your shoulders. Exhale as you lift; inhale as you lower.

BACK

Position A   Position B

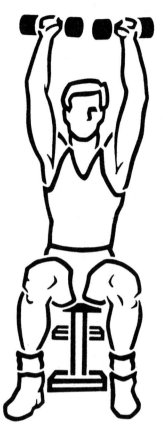

MILITARY PRESSES Hold dumb-bells above your shoulders, level with the ears. Arms will be L-shaped with shoulders relaxed. Slowly raise the bells straight up until arms are fully extended, but elbows are not locked. Do not arch your back or elevate your shoulders. Exhale as you lift and inhale as you lower the weights.

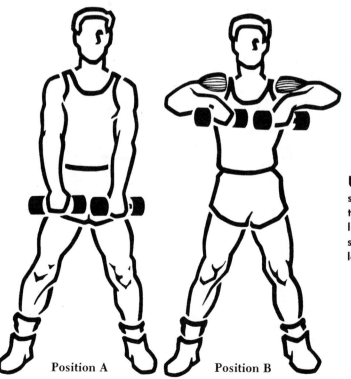

UPRIGHT ROWS Stand with your feet slightly farther than shoulder-width apart, knees slightly bent. Hold weights in front of thighs and lean forward slightly to avoid arching your back when you lift. With shoulders relaxed, bend your elbows to lift the dumbbells straight up to your collarbone. Exhale as you lift and inhale as you lower the bells.

Position A   Position B

SHOULDERS

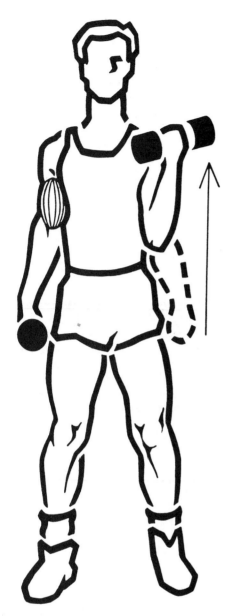

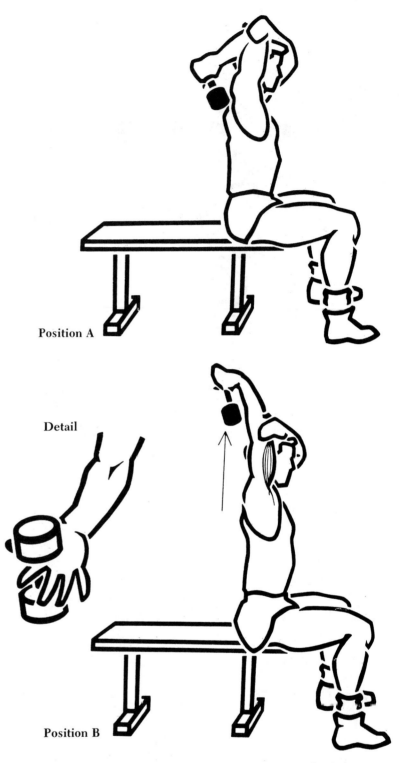

Position A

Detail

Position B

ALTERNATE CURLS Stand with your feet slightly farther than shoulder width apart and knees slightly bent. Hold weights at your sides and lean forward slightly to avoid arching your back when you lift. Keeping shoulders down and elbows at your side, raise the forearm only to lift the weight to the shoulder. Lift one dumbbell at a time, alternating sides.

ARMS

FRENCH CURLS Sit with feet apart and back straight, but not arched. Hold the end of the dumbbell in one hand (see detail) and use the other hand to steady the weight-bearing arm so the elbow remains pointing straight up near the ear. Raise your forearm overhead without locking the elbow, exhaling on the lift and inhaling as the dumbbell lowers behind your head. Be careful that the weight-bearing arm does not shift back and forth.

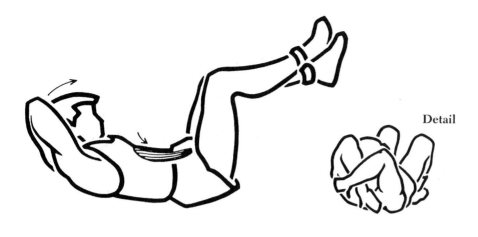

Detail

CRUNCHES Lie on your back on a cushioned surface with knees bent. Cross your forearms behind your head so that fingertips touch opposite shoulders. This creates a cradle where your head rests. Elevate your legs until they form an L, with thighs perpendicular to the floor and lower legs parallel to it, then cross your ankles. Slowly raise your upper back, using the abdominal muscles, and not straining the neck, then pull your upper torso toward your legs. Exhale as you lift and inhale as you lower.

Position A   Position B

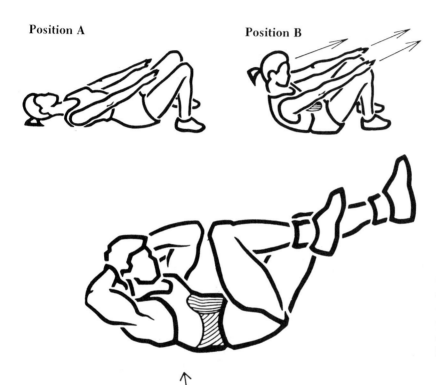

CURL-UPS Lie on your back on a cushioned surface with lower legs at about a 90-degree angle with the floor and feet hip-width apart. Extend arms in front. Raise only your head and shoulders until the upper back is off the floor and your fingertips are on the thighs. Slide your fingers in a path along your thighs to the middle of your kneecaps, then lower your shoulders back to the floor. Exhale as you curl up and inhale as you return to the floor.

BICYCLES Lie on your back on a cushioned surface with hands behind head. Lift both legs into an L shape, keeping the lower leg parallel to the floor during the exercise. Raise your shoulders from the mat and alternately touch an elbow to the opposite knee while moving your thighs slightly back and forth. Keep your lower back pressed into the mat and contract your abdominal muscles to support the action. Touching the elbow to both sides is 1 repetition.

POPS Lie on your back, hands next to hips, palms down, legs straight up with knees slightly bent and ankles crossed. As you exhale, raise the buttocks one inch, then inhale as you lower the buttocks. Don't drop the hips sharply, but move slowly and steadily.

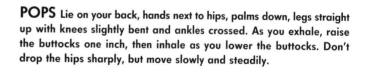

ABDOMINALS

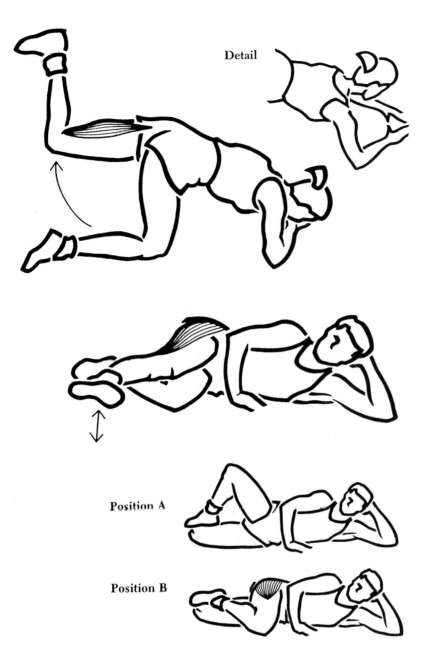

Detail

KNEE-UPS Rest on your elbows and knees with hands touching to form a triangle where your head can rest. Raise one leg until your thigh is parallel to the floor. The lower leg forms an L-shaped 90-degree angle. Keep your foot flexed so toes do not point. Lower this leg to the knee of the supporting leg as you inhale and raise it to hip level as you exhale.

OUTER THIGH LIFTS Lie on your side supporting the head with one hand while the other hand rests on the mat in front of your chest for balance. The leg against the floor should bend at the knee at a 45-degree angle, while the upper leg extends straight out from the body parallel with the thigh of the lower leg. Keeping your foot flexed so that the toes do *not* point, inhale as you lower the extended leg to the floor and exhale as you raise it to hip level.

CORKSCREWS Lie on your side with your head resting on one hand while the other supports your body by resting on the mat in front of your chest. Place the foot of your upper leg on the knee of the lower leg (as you get stronger, the foot will hang just above the knee). Slowly lower the knee of the upper leg toward the floor while you inhale, and return the knee as you exhale.

INNER THIGH LIFTS Lie on your side with one foot beneath a bench or chair and the upper foot resting on the chair or bench seat. Rest your head on one hand, place the other in front of your chest for balance. Exhale as you lift the lower leg to touch the bottom of the bench; inhale as you lower the leg to the floor. Raise and lower the leg with control.

Position A

Position B

▶ You have a choice of exercises.
Refer to your strength program chart.

LEGS

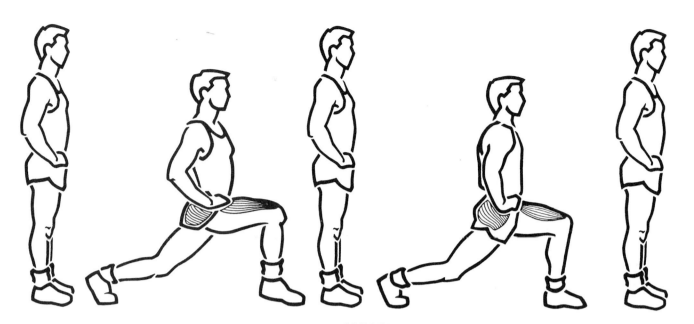

LUNGE WALKS

Begin with feet together and hands on hips. You may want to practice the first few sessions with one hand on a wall for balance and control. Keeping your torso erect throughout the exercise, take a giant step forward (two and a half to three feet), and transfer your weight to the forward leg, keeping the heel of the front foot on the ground. The back leg bends slightly and the heel raises, but the knee never touches the ground. Sink until the thigh of the front leg is parallel to the ground. Exhale as you bring the rear leg forward and stand up straight with feet together. Take a giant step forward with the opposite leg, sink, then bring feet together again.

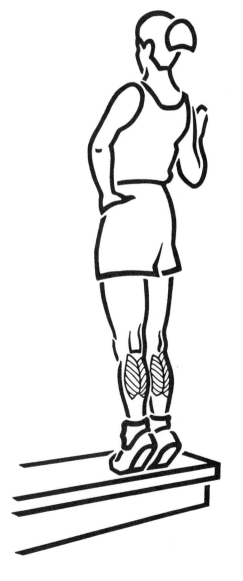

CALF RAISES

Stand next to a wall using one hand for balance, with the balls of your feet together on a step or thick telephone book. Keeping knees straight but not locked, inhale as you slowly lower your heels toward the floor and exhale as you rise on the balls of your feet. Be sure that your ankles do not twist outward.

Cool-Down Stretches

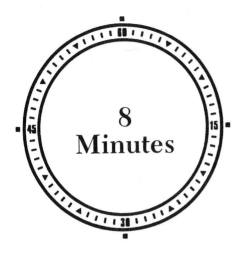

8
Minutes

Lower Body

The Cool-Down stretches that end your workout are different than the stretches that began it. Follow them in the sequence shown.

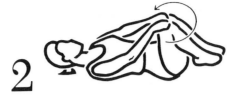

2

KNEE CIRCLES (for lower back) Slide hands onto kneecaps and circle knees to the right 4 times, keeping abdominals pressed into the lower back so that the base of the spine is against the mat. Gradually make the circles smaller, then reverse the direction for 4 more circles, gradually making the circles larger.

● Transition: Keep one leg toward your chest and extend the other leg straight out along the mat, with the foot flexed so your toes point to the ceiling.

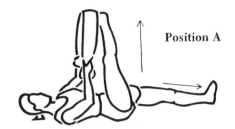

Position A

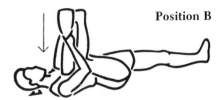

Position B

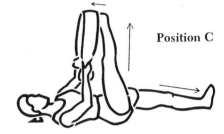

Position C

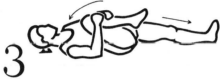

3

THIGH TO CHEST (for lower back) With hands clasped below the knee of the bent leg, exhale as you pull the thigh up and back toward your shoulder. Don't push down toward the ground, but gently pull in an arc toward the shoulder.

● Transition: Keep thigh in the same position, with the other leg still stretched out.

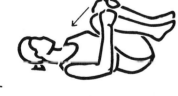

1

THE TORTOISE (for lower back) Lie on your back on the exercise mat and lift knees toward the chest with hands grasping the lower leg beneath the knee. Lengthen your neck and look straight up. Inhale through the nose and exhale through the mouth.

● Transition: Stay in the same position.

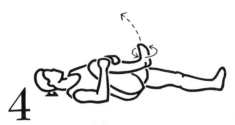

4

FOOT CIRCLES (for ankle) Circle the ankle of the bent leg 4 times to the right, then 4 times to the left.

● Transition: Wrap either a towel or your hands around the ball of the same foot.

5

BOW AND ARROW (for back of leg) Press your heel straight up to the ceiling until the leg is almost straight, but do not lock the knee. Keep your foot flat and the leg extended as you hold the stretch and exhale. Inhale as you bend the knee while using the towel or your hands to help to bring the thigh to your chest, forming a 90-degree angle. The sole of the foot faces the ceiling. Then exhale as you press the heel straight up once more. Throughout these stretches, the leg on the floor is extended.

● Transition: Slowly bring your thigh down to your chest, and put aside the towel. Place the foot of this leg on the knee of your outstretched leg.

Position A   Position B

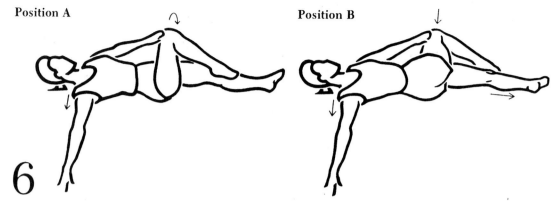

6

BACK TWIST (for back) Grasp the outside of the bent knee with the opposite hand. Stretch the other hand away from the body, level with the shoulder. Gently push the bent leg toward the floor while keeping your shoulders square on the mat. Exhale as you gently press downward, and inhale as you hold the stretch for at least 30 seconds. Use 3 or more exhalations to relax the leg toward the floor. Finally, turn the head away from the direction of the twist.

● Transition: Release the stretch and straighten your head.

7

KNEE TOUCH (for back) With both hands, grasp beneath the knee. Lift your head, neck, and upper back from the floor and touch your kneecap with your nose.

● Transition: Return your head, upper body, and bent leg to the mat.

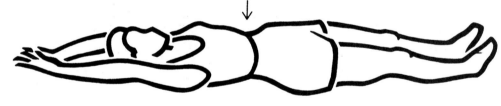

8

FULL-BODY STRETCH (for all major muscles) Stretch your arms overhead and extend both legs as you exhale. Press abdominals toward the floor to keep lower back flat.

 ● First Transition: Start the series with *Thigh to Chest* on the other side.

● Second Transition: After completing the series on the opposite side through *Full-Body Stretch*, roll over onto your stomach.

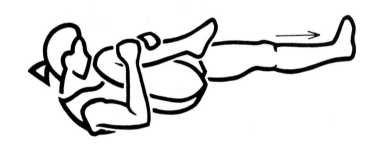

9

THIGH PULL (for top of thigh) Lying on your stomach, take hold of the foot with the hand on the same side of the body and pull the lower leg and foot to the buttocks. Do each side.

 ● Transition: Release your grasp on the foot and place both hands under the shoulders with forearms flat on the floor, and head looking down at the mat.

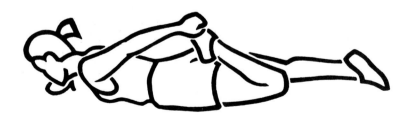

Cool-Down Stretches Continue

Cool-Down Stretches

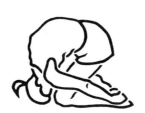

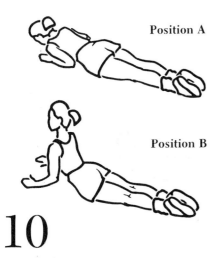

Position A

Position B

10

COBRA (for back and abdominals) Pressing the palms of the hands into the floor lift the upper body, without collapsing the shoulders, using the bent forearms to raise the torso while pelvis remains on the floor.
* Transition: Lower your torso until you are flat on the mat. Push yourself up until you are sitting on knees and feet.

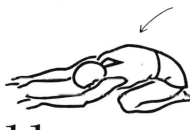

11

SLEEPING CAT (for lower back) Exhale as you bend from the waist and extend your arms out in front of you until your chest is on your thighs.
* Transition: Raise your torso and rest on hands and knees.

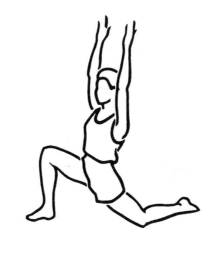

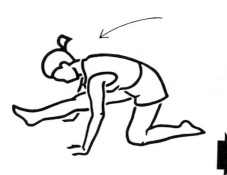

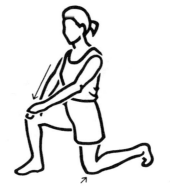

12

RABBIT (for upper back and top of shoulders) Place the crown of your head, the baby's "soft spot," onto the floor, as close to your knees as possible. Firmly wrap the palms of your hands around the soles of your arches. Deeply inhale, then exhale as you slowly lift the buttocks into the air while the arms straighten. You will feel this stretch in the upper shoulders.
* Transition: Roll upright until your torso is erect and hands are next to the knees.

13

MODIFIED LUNGE (for front of leg) Using the muscles in your thighs, move one foot forward until the knee is perpendicular to the floor and in line with the heel. Move the pelvis forward to stretch the back leg. The back thigh should form a 45-degree angle with the floor, and the top of the foot should be flat against the mat. Adjust your front foot to keep the knee over the toe. Raise your hands over your head, keeping the torso erect as you exhale. If you need to stabilize your balance place both hands on the front knee, then repeat the stretch on the other side.
* Transition: Inhale as your pelvis moves backward to straighten your forward leg, and place your hands either on your knee or on the mat for balance.

14

FORWARD BOW (for back of leg) Bending from the waist, exhale as you lower your chest toward your thigh. Be sure you are not sitting back, but that your stabilizing knee is directly under the hip, and your buttocks are over the knee.
* Transition: Bend the stretching leg so you are on your knees and start the *Modified Lunge* and *Forward Bow* on the other side.

15

VERTICAL RISE (to protect back upon standing) Bring the front foot back so that your thigh parallels the floor. Place both hands on top of the knee in front of you, and pull the toes of your rear foot forward. Press down on the knee, stabilizing your balance as you stand up.

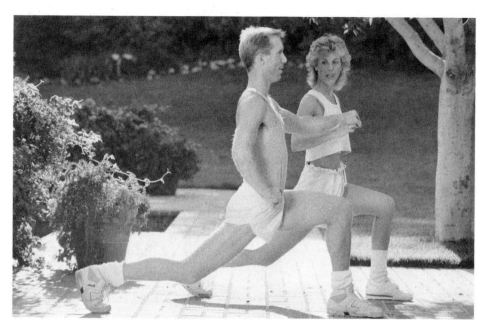

Take the Challenge

Experiencing movement for personal pleasure, along with the noticeable changes in your body, have hopefully encouraged you to make activity a regular part of your week. Try joining a 5K race, sign up for a rafting trip, or prepare for a trek in the United States or Europe. By trying a new adventure and mixing the activities you choose, you'll maintain a fitness challenge—and your enthusiasm for life.

It's time to compare your progress, so turn to the Appendix and take your fitness tests and measurements at the end of this program. If you have worked your way up, beginning with *The Gain Program,* your six months of hard work should show a noticeably new you. Those who started five months ago in *The Train Program* have the benefit of getting off the resolution treadmill and on with an exercise lifestyle. If you entered *Full Circle Fitness* as a moderate exerciser, your four months on *The Maintain Program* have brought structure and measurable progress to your best intentions.

Give yourself a hug! You have accomplished a purposeful exercise plan in just four to six months and you have begun a lifetime investment in your own well-being. Now you can graduate to lifestyle exercise with either *A Handle on Health* or *The Competitive Edge.* If, however, you wish to plateau your activity at any of the programs without progressing immediately to the next, you will still realize many of the health benefits of regular exercise.

Little victories become major milestones, so before you begin the next three chapters—celebrate life!

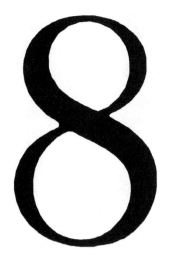

When you are ready for A Handle on Health, you have been exercising two or three times per week for six months and scored in the upper ranges on the fitness assessments.

A HANDLE ON HEALTH

Philosophers say that you can only truly possess something once you let it go. At first that belief doesn't seem to make any sense. But I've noticed that most clients tend to follow a pattern. Somewhat reluctantly they begin to exercise, then newfound success turns them into fitness fanatics who build their lives around exercise. They buy wardrobes of designer sweats, endlessly monitor each increment of muscle development, and brag about the regularity of their aerobics.

Interestingly, it's the people who never leave the fanatic stage who tend to stop exercising altogether. They burn out and leap to another avid hobby. Those who finally "let go" of that compulsiveness and allow exercise and rational eating to become part of the everyday humdrum routines are the ones who keep exercising. And they are the ones who receive the lifetime mental and physical benefits.

A Handle on Health was created to be a comfortable program that integrates well with your daily routines. It will help you maintain your weight, modify health risks, and relieve stress. You've learned the fundamentals of a *Full Circle Fitness* exercise prescription, so now your challenge is to stay interested and make activity rewarding. To maximize your effort, I'll be introducing different methods for the strength routine. You'll also add 30 minutes of aerobic training on two extra days which totals four hours a week for health maintenance.

As Olympic contenders know, there is always something to work on even if you do the same exercise every day, for the rest of your life. Your past successes prove its value. And with *A Handle on Health*, you can achieve optimal health and feel the rewards.

Training Tips For A Handle on Health

Maintain your exercise schedule and reasonable eating. Too many skipped sessions, and you start spiralling downward. Remember, it takes two weeks to lose what it took six weeks to gain.

Try new approaches to keep exercise interesting. Go to a new aerobics class, try a stationary bike, find a training buddy, go hiking!

Investigate opportunities for sports participation. Many charities now sponsor 5K and 10K races, aerobics classes, and short bicycle events. They offer a nonstress situation for good causes.

Recognize that you are scheduling only four hours of exercise each week. That's a time commitment you should be able to keep.

Make exercising a convenience. Explore the possibility of buying equipment for a home gym.

Turn vacations into fitness adventures. Go cross-country skiing, bike touring, river rafting, or canoeing. Many companies now offer this type of tour.

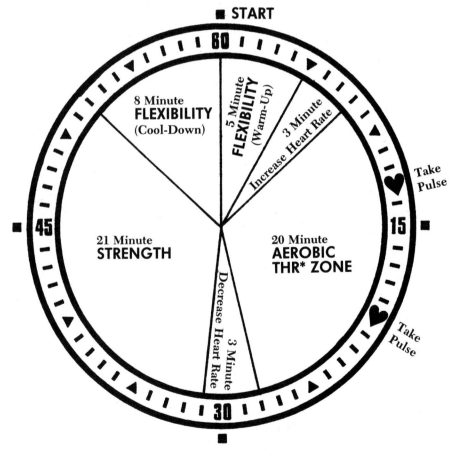

A Handle on Health Exercise Hour

**1 Hour Workout 3 Times per Week and
30 Minutes of Aerobic Exercise 2 Days a Week**

Training Heart Rate

Warm-Up Stretches

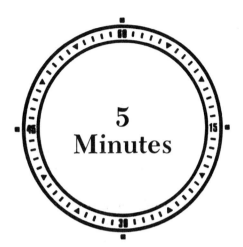

5 Minutes

Equipment

A mat or folded quilt and old bath towel.

Secrets of Stretching

● Warm up your muscles before stretching.
● Exhale as you stretch and inhale as you move into the next position.
● Stretch until you feel tension, then hold the position for 10 to 30 seconds.
● Avoid bouncing.
● Be precise when moving into position.
● Move smoothly and leisurely and *breathe*.
● Perform the stretches in the order listed.

Lower Body

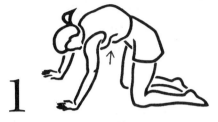

1

CAT AND CAMEL (for lower, middle, and upper back) Rest on hands and knees, making sure that the knees are under the hips and the hands are directly under the shoulders. As you exhale, round your spine, curling the torso away from the mat, and press your stomach toward the back. Inhale as you lift your head and gently lower the pelvis. Don't overarch your back. Exhale as you round the spine again. Alternate these 3 times.
● Transition: Return to starting position.

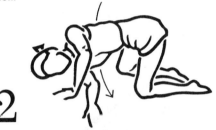

2

BACK BRIDGE (for middle back) Roll one shoulder onto the mat while both knees remain on the floor. Keep the knees under your hips and extend one arm, palm up, under the bridge formed by your body. Push into the shoulder with the arm that is stabilizing the bridge so that you feel the stretch between the shoulder blade and the spine. Exhale as you intensify the stretch, then repeat on the other side.
● Transition: Straighten your shoulders, then return to sitting on your heels.

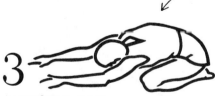

3

SLEEPING CAT (for lower back) Exhale as you bend from the waist and extend your arms out in front of you until your chest is on your thighs.
● Transition: Firmly wrap the palms of your hands around the soles of your arches.

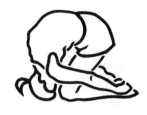

4

RABBIT (for upper back and top of shoulders) Place the crown of your head, the baby's "soft spot," onto the floor, as close to your knees as possible. Deeply inhale, then exhale as you slowly lift the buttocks into the air while the arms straighten. You will feel this stretch in the upper shoulders.
● Transition: Roll upright until your torso is erect and hands are next to the knees.

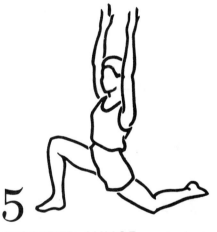

5

MODIFIED LUNGE (for front of leg) Using the muscles in your thighs, move one foot forward until the knee is perpendicular to the floor and in line with the heel. Move the pelvis forward to stretch the back leg. The back thigh should form a 45-degree angle with the floor, and the top of the foot should be flat against the mat. Adjust your front foot to keep the knee over the toe. Raise your hands over your head, keeping the torso erect as you exhale. If you need to stabilize your balance place both hands on the front knee.
● Transition: Inhale as your pelvis moves backward to straighten your forward leg, and place your hands either on your knee or on the mat for balance.

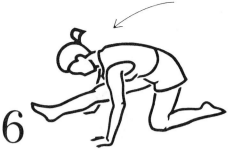

6

FORWARD BOW (for back of leg)
Bending from the waist, exhale as you lower your chest toward your thigh. Be sure you are not sitting back, but that your stabilizing knee is directly under the hip, and your buttocks are over the knee.

● First Transition: Pull back the forward leg to bring both knees together. Start the series with *The Modified Lunge* on the other side.

● Second Transition: After completing the series on the opposite side through the *Forward Bow* pull back the forward leg to bring both knees under you.

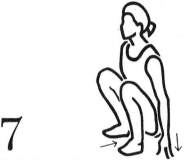

7

DO THE DUCK (for ankles and calf)
With hands on either side, shift your weight until feet are shoulder-width apart and flat on the ground. Maintain the position while you stretch the lower leg.

● Transition: Shift weight to your knees.

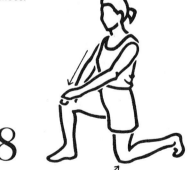

8

VERTICAL RISE (to protect back upon standing) Bring one foot forward so that your thigh parallels the floor. Place both hands on top of the knee in front of you, and pull the toes of your rear foot forward. Press down on the knee, stabilizing your balance as you stand up.

Upper Body

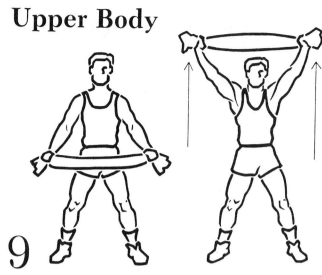

9

SHOULDER ARCH (for shoulders) Taking the towel in both hands, stand with your feet farther than shoulder-width apart with arms straight. Without locking your elbows, raise both your arms in an arc, keeping the towel taut, until hands swing behind the head. Lower your hands to the thighs and repeat the movement smoothly 5 times.

● Transition: Hold the last stretch above the head and bend the knees slightly.

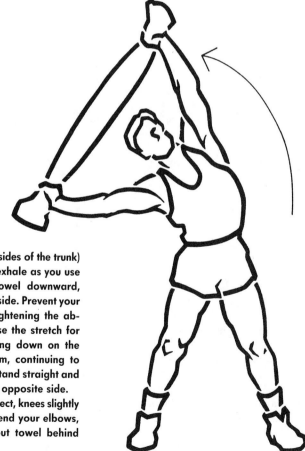

10

SIDE STRETCH (for sides of the trunk)
Keeping the towel taut, exhale as you use one hand to pull the towel downward, bending the trunk to one side. Prevent your back from arching by tightening the abdominal muscles. Increase the stretch for 3 deep breaths by pulling down on the towel with the lower arm, continuing to bend to the side. Slowly stand straight and repeat the stretch on the opposite side.

● Transition: Stand erect, knees slightly bent, towel over head. Bend your elbows, lowering the stretched-out towel behind your head.

Warm-Up Stretches Continue

Warm-Up Stretches
Upper Body

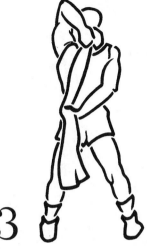

13

ARM PULL (for back of arm) Bring your free arm behind your back to grab the towel at a comfortable distance. The arm holding the towel should be near the ear with the elbow pointing forward. Pull down on the towel to stretch the back of the bent arm as you exhale. Hold the stretch for 3 deep breaths, keeping the tension in the towel constant. Then switch the towel to the other hand and repeat the stretch.

●   Transition: Let go of the towel with the upper arm and extend both arms downward with palms facing toward the rear. Grasp both ends and stretch the towel behind your back.

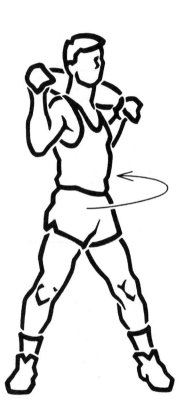

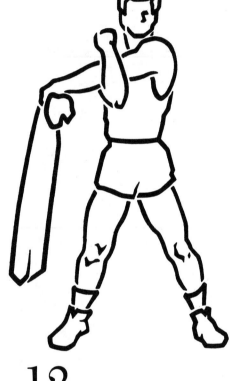

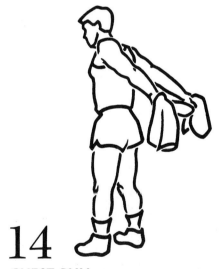

11

WAIST TWISTS (for back and trunk) With toes and hips pointing straight ahead and abdominals tightened, anchor your hips by pressing the abdominal muscles toward the back. Twist your trunk slowly in one direction as far as you can without letting the hips turn. Hold the towel in a straight line to keep your elbows back, and face forward. Twist to the opposite side, then alternate sides 8 times.

●   Transition: Face forward and release your grip from one end of the towel.

12

SHOULDER PULL (for shoulder) Extend the hand holding the towel straight in front of you. Your free hand, palm up, travels under the extended arm and hooks around the upper arm just above the elbow. Use the hooked arm to pull the straight arm toward the middle of your body. Hold for 3 breaths, then transfer the towel to the other hand and repeat the stretch on that side.

●   Transition: Bring the hand holding the towel over your head, then bend your elbow so the towel is hanging to the floor behind you.

14

CHEST PULL (for chest) Holding the towel in a straight line, lift both arms straight up until you feel the stretch in the chest and shoulder muscles. Take 3 deep breaths in this position while the muscles relax.

Aerobic Conditioning

Activity Swim, walk, cycle, rowing machine, dance exercise, cross-country ski machine, jog, run, or a combination of these.

Intensity **3 minutes** to elevate heart rate—**20 minutes** in your personal heart rate zone—**3 minutes** to decrease heart rate to 100–110 beats per minute

The Heart Rate Chart

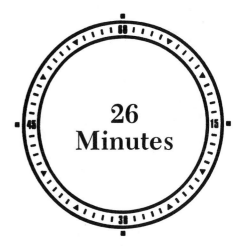

Aerobic Training Tips

- Monitor your exercise intensity twice during each aerobic workout: Take your pulse at 8 minutes and 15 minutes into the activity.
- Take the time to learn the proper form and method for each activity.
- Move continuously for at least 20 minutes.
- If you exercise outdoors, accommodate to the weather.

beats per minute—10-second count

Round Up to Nearest Age and Resting Heart Rate		(RPE Scale) 11–15
Age	Resting Heart Rate	Handle on Health 60–80%
20 years	60	144–172 **24–29**
	70	148–174 **25–29**
	80	152–176 **25–29**
30 years	60	138–164 **23–27**
	70	142–166 **24–28**
	80	146–168 **24–28**
40 years	60	132–156 **22–26**
	70	136–158 **23–26**
	80	140–160 **23–27**
50 years	60	126–148 **21–25**
	70	130–150 **22–25**
	80	134–152 **22–25**
60+ years	60	120–140 **20–23**
	70	124–142 **21–24**
	80	128–144 **21–24**

Strength Training

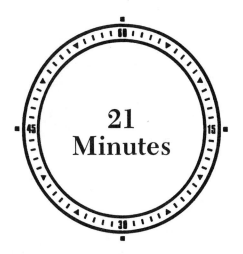

21 Minutes

Equipment

- 8- to 12-pound dumbbells for women
- 2–5-pound ankle weights
- 10- to 15-pound dumbbells for men
- Flat exercise bench
- "Record your Workout" chart

Strength Training Secrets

- Pay attention to the execution of each exercise.
- Concentrate on the muscles you are using.
- Exhale on the contraction—the lift or push—and inhale during the opposite movement.
- Use slow, fully controlled movements in both directions without permitting momentum to do any of the work.
- Move through the complete range of motion that you can achieve.
- Sets are a defined number of repetitions done consecutively (i.e., 1–2 sets, or times).
- Keep exercises in the indicated sequence.
- Work up to 15 repetitions, then increase the weight of dumbbells by 2 pounds every 4 weeks.

A Handle on Health

CHEST
1. **Chest Presses,** dumbbells, 8 reps × 2 sets
2. **Flyes,** dumbbells, 8 reps × 2 sets

BACK
1. **One-Arm Rows,** dumbbells, 8 reps × 2 sets
2. **Double Rows,** dumbbells, 8 reps × 2 sets

SHOULDERS
1. **Military Presses,** dumbbells, 8 reps × 2 sets
2. **Upright Rows,** dumbbells, 8 reps × 2 sets

ARMS
1. **Alternate Curls,** dumbbells, 8 reps × 2 sets
2. **Concentration Curls,** dumbbells, 8 reps × 2 sets
3. **Dips,** 8 reps × 2 sets
4. **Kickbacks,** dumbbells, 8 reps × 2 sets

ABDOMINALS
1. **Crunches,** 24 reps × 2 sets
2. **Side Crunches,** (each side) 24 reps × 1 set
3. **Bicycles,** 24 reps × 2 sets
4. **Pops,** 24 reps × 2 sets

LEGS
1. **Knee-ups,** ankle weight, 32 reps × 1 set (each leg)
2. **Outer Thigh Lifts,** ankle weight, 32 reps × 1 set (each leg)
3. **Corkscrews,** ankle weight, 32 reps × 1 set (each leg)
4. **Inner Thigh Lifts,** ankle weight, 32 reps × 1 set (each leg)
or
1. **Lunge Walks,** 24 reps × 2 sets
2. **Sissy Squats,** 16 reps × 2 sets
   and
3. **Calf Raises,** 24 reps × 2 sets

● Do the first set of each exercise until you work through the whole body, then repeat the whole routine with a heavier weight for the second set. Each exercise is done for 2 sets.

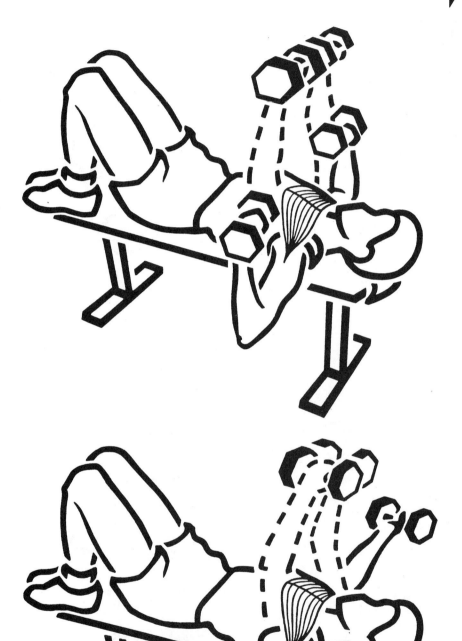

CHEST PRESSES Lie on your back on an exercise bench (a narrow sturdy coffee table or two ottomans pushed together will work) with feet on the bench, knees bent to keep your back flat, and dumbbells in both hands. Raise the dumbbells straight from the shoulder until arms are extended but elbows remain slightly bent. Inhale as you slowly lower the dumbbells to chest level, always keeping the forearms straight up at a 90-degree angle to the bench. Exhale as you push the bells overhead.

FLYES Lie on an exercise bench with knees bent and feet on the bench to keep your back flat. Hold dumbbells over your chest with hands together, keeping your elbows slightly bent. As you inhale, lower the bells in a circular arc until they are level with your chest. Your elbows should be pointing to the floor but not lower than your wrists. Exhale as you raise the dumbbells to bring them together over your chest.

CHEST

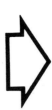

• Do the first set of each exercise until you work through the whole body, then repeat the whole routine with a heavier weight for the second set. Each exercise is done for 2 sets.

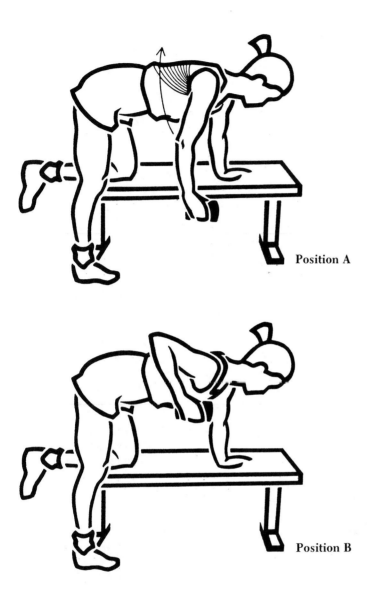

Position A

Position B

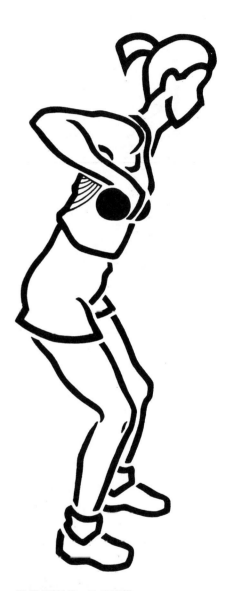

ONE-ARM ROWS Rest the arm and leg of one side on a low bench holding a dumbbell in the free hand. Keeping your shoulder immobile and your back flat, raise the weight straight up along the side of your body to just below the armpit. Exhale as you lift the bell, inhale as you lower it.

BACK

DOUBLE ROWS Bend forward slightly from the waist with knees bent and feet shoulder-width apart. With a weight in each hand, let your arms hang relaxed at your sides, palms facing to the rear. Keep your back straight as you raise the weights to your armpits *without* lifting your shoulders. Exhale as you lift; inhale as you lower.

Position A   Position B

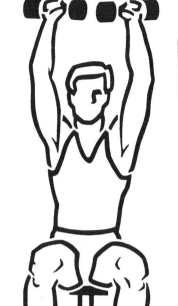

For Circuit Weight Training

● Do the first set of each exercise until you work through the whole body, then repeat the whole routine with a heavier weight for the second set. Each exercise is done for 2 sets.

MILITARY PRESSES Hold dumbbells above your shoulders, level with the ears. Arms will be L-shaped with shoulders relaxed. Slowly raise the bells straight up until arms are fully extended, but elbows are not locked. Do not arch your back or elevate your shoulders. Exhale as you lift and inhale as you lower the weights.

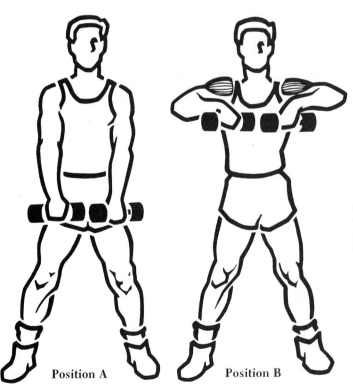

UPRIGHT ROWS Stand with your feet slightly farther than shoulder-width apart, knees slightly bent. Hold weights in front of thighs and lean forward slightly to avoid arching your back when you lift. With shoulders relaxed, bend your elbows to lift the dumbbells straight up to your collarbone. Exhale as you lift and inhale as you lower the bells.

SHOULDERS

Position A   Position B

For Circuit Weight Training

● Do the first set of each exercise until you work through the whole body, then repeat the whole routine with a heavier weight for the second set. Each exercise is done for 2 sets.

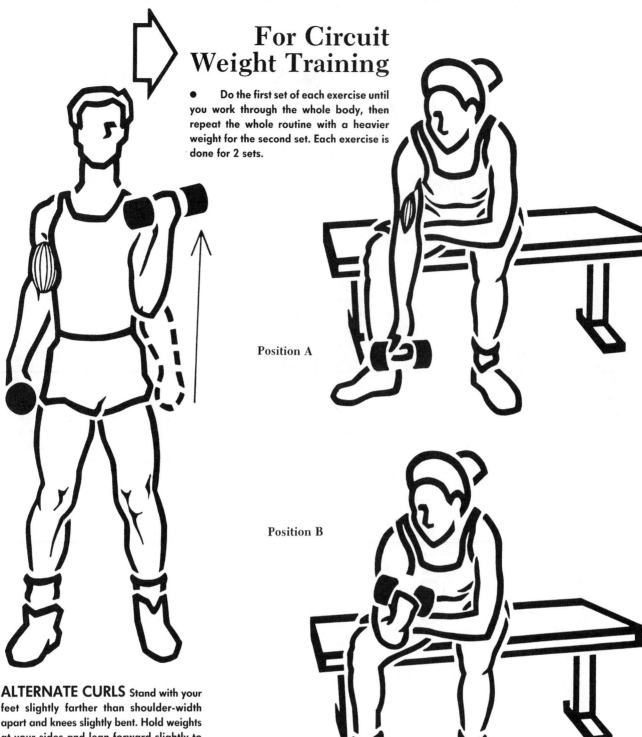

Position A

Position B

ALTERNATE CURLS Stand with your feet slightly farther than shoulder-width apart and knees slightly bent. Hold weights at your sides and lean forward slightly to avoid arching your back when you lift. Keeping shoulders down and elbows at your side, raise the forearm only to lift the weight to the shoulder. Lift one dumbbell at a time, alternating sides.

CONCENTRATION CURLS Sit on a bench or chair. Leaning forward from the hips with a straight back, place one hand on the opposite knee. With the other hand, grasp a dumbbell and let your arm hang straight and relaxed. As you exhale, raise the weight by bending your elbow. Be sure that the shoulder doesn't drop and that the effort is felt in the arm, not the shoulder. Inhale as you lower the weight.

ARMS

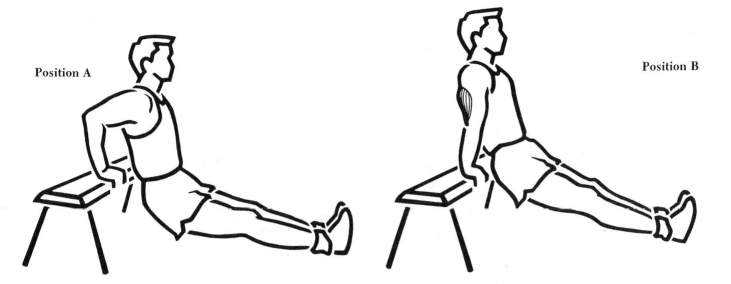

Position A

Position B

DIPS Sit on the edge of a sturdy chair or bench, with legs together and hands resting on the seat next to your buttocks. Support your upper body with your hands and step forward, one foot at a time, so that both legs are extended fully and your weight is balanced on your heels. Keeping your back straight and shoulders down, slowly lower your body until the upper arm is parallel to the floor and elbows point straight behind you. Keep the body close to the bench. Inhale as you lower and exhale as you push back up.

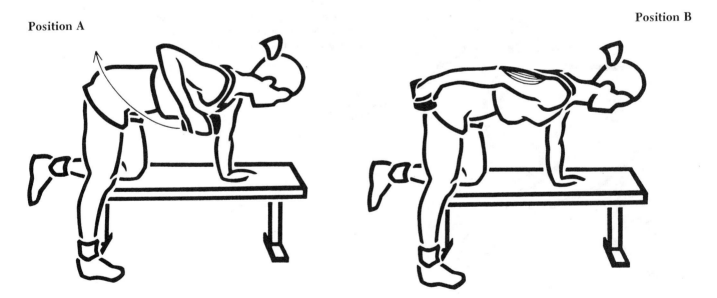

Position A

Position B

KICKBACKS Rest your knee and hand on a chair or bench. Keeping the back straight, grasp a dumbbell in the opposite hand and bring your elbow to waist level so the upper arm is at your side and the forearm hangs straight down. Keeping the upper arm immobile, exhale as you extend the lower arm in a straight line behind you. Bend your elbow to bring the weight to your shoulder and then extend it behind you again. Be sure that your wrist stays straight in line with the lower arm.

CRUNCHES Lie on your back on a cushioned surface with knees bent. Cross your forearms behind your head (see detail) so that fingertips touch opposite shoulders. This creates a cradle where your head rests. Elevate your legs until they form an L, with thighs perpendicular to the floor and lower legs parallel to it, then cross your ankles. Slowly raise your upper back, using the abdominal muscles, and not straining the neck, then pull your upper torso toward your legs. Exhale as you lift and inhale as you lower.

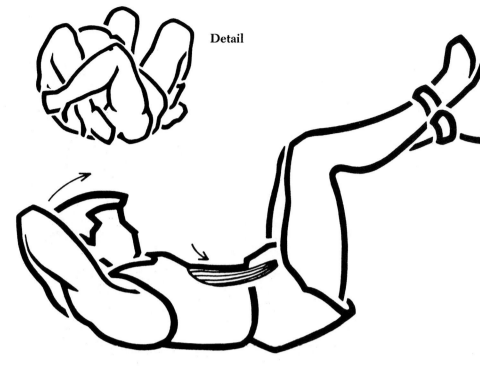

Detail

SIDE CRUNCHES Lie on your back with knees bent. Cross legs at the knee, then let them fall gently, in one unit, to one side. Lift your head and shoulders with arms reaching in the opposite direction from your legs. Roll up with straight arms, slowly exhaling as you reach diagonally. Do not roll all the way down. For circuit weight training do one side on the first set and the other side for the second set.

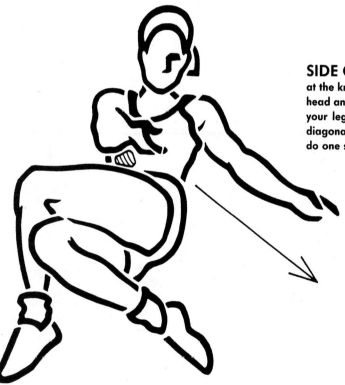

ABDOMINALS

▶ For circuit weight training, do one set of each exercise per circuit.

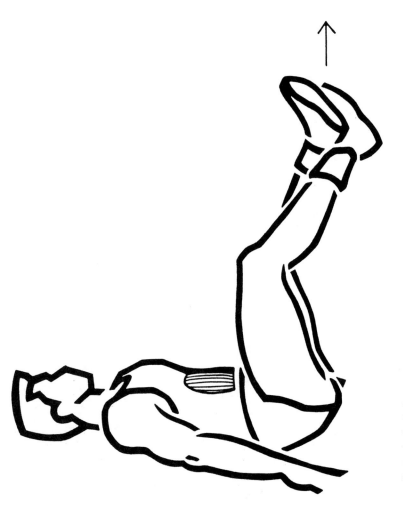

BICYCLES Lie on your back on a cushioned surface with hands behind head. Lift both legs into an L-shape, keeping the lower leg parallel to the floor during the exercise. Raise your shoulders from the mat and alternately touch an elbow to the opposite knee while moving your thighs slightly back and forth. Keep your lower back pressed into the mat and contract your abdominal muscles to support the action. Touching the elbow to both sides is 1 repetition.

POPS Lie on your back, hands next to hips, palms down, legs straight up with knees slightly bent and ankles crossed. As you exhale, raise the buttocks one inch, then inhale as you lower the buttocks. Don't drop the hips sharply, but move slowly and steadily.

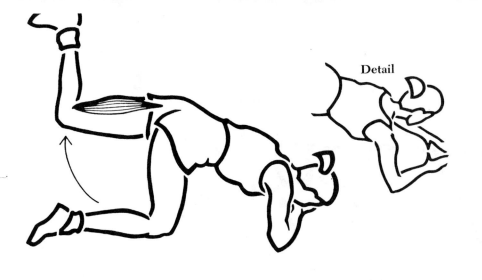

Detail

KNEE-UPS Rest on your elbows and knees with hands touching to form a triangle where your head can rest. Raise one leg until your thigh is parallel to the floor. The lower leg forms an L-shaped 90-degree angle. Keep your foot flexed so toes do not point. Lower this leg to the knee of the supporting leg as you inhale and raise it to hip level as you exhale.

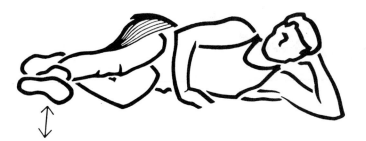

OUTER THIGH LIFTS Lie on your side supporting the head with one hand while the other hand rests on the mat in front of your chest for balance. The leg against the floor should bend at the knee at a 45-degree angle, while the upper leg extends straight out from the body parallel with the thigh of the lower leg. Keeping your foot flexed so that the toes do *not* point, inhale as you lower the extended leg to the floor and exhale as you raise it to hip level.

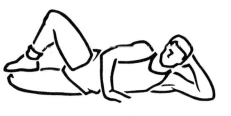

Position A   Position B

CORKSCREWS Lie on your side with your head resting on one hand while the other supports your body by resting on the mat in front of your chest. Place the foot of your upper leg on the knee of the lower leg (as you get stronger, the foot will hang just above the knee). Slowly lower the knee of the upper leg toward the floor while you inhale, and return the knee as you exhale.

▶ You have a choice of exercises.
Refer to your strength program chart.

INNER THIGH LIFTS Lie on your side with one foot beneath a bench or chair and the upper foot resting on the chair or bench seat. Rest your head on one hand, place the other in front of your chest for balance. Exhale as you lift the lower leg to touch the bottom of the bench; inhale as you lower the leg to the floor. Raise and lower the leg with control.

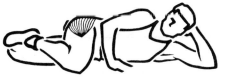

LEGS

▶ For circuit weight training, do one side, then other side as a second set.

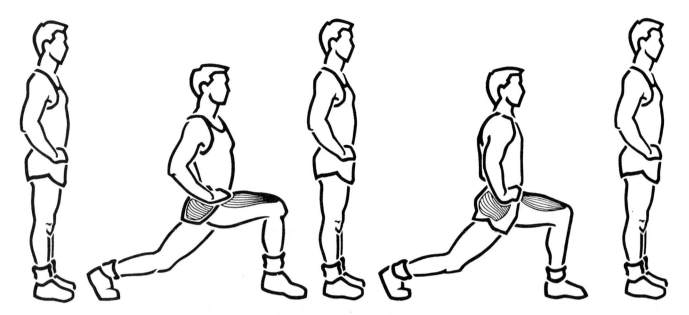

LUNGE WALKS Begin with feet together and hands on hips. You may want to practice the first few sessions with one hand on a wall for balance and control. Keeping your torso erect throughout the exercise, take a giant step forward (two and a half to three feet), and transfer your weight to the forward leg, keeping the heel of the front foot on the ground. The back leg bends slightly and the heel raises, but the knee never touches the ground. Sink until the thigh of the front leg is parallel to the ground. Exhale as you bring the rear leg forward and stand up straight with feet together. Take a giant step forward with the opposite leg, sink, then bring feet together again.

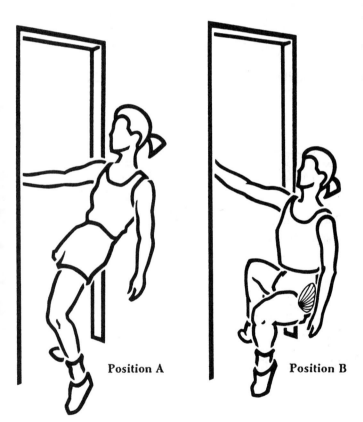

Position A   Position B

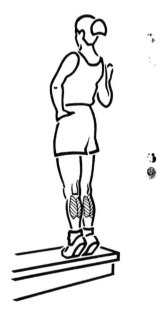

SISSY SQUATS Stand at a doorway on the balls of your feet shoulder-width apart and toes pointed outward. Hold onto the door jamb at shoulder height and lean back the length of your arm. Bend your knees, lowering your buttocks halfway to the floor as you inhale. Push the pelvis toward the door, squeezing the buttocks, as you exhale.

CALF RAISES Stand next to a wall using one hand for balance, with the balls of your feet together on a step or thick telephone book. Keeping knees straight but not locked, inhale as you slowly lower your heels toward the floor and exhale as you rise on the balls of your feet. Be sure that your ankles do not twist outward.

Cool-Down Stretches

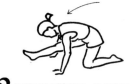

8 Minutes

The Cool-Down stretches that end your workout are the same as the stretches that began it—except you'll do them in opposite order. These illustrations show the correct flow. For instructions on how to perform them, turn to pages 94 to 96.

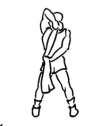

5 ARM PULL

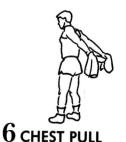

6 CHEST PULL

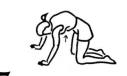

7 CAT AND CAMEL

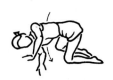

8 BACK BRIDGE
Repeat on the Other Side

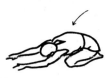

9 SLEEPING CAT

10 RABBIT

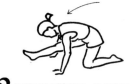

11 MODIFIED LUNGE

12 FORWARD BOW
Repeat on the Other Side
Start With Modified Lunge

13 DO THE DUCK

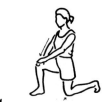

14 VERTICAL RISE

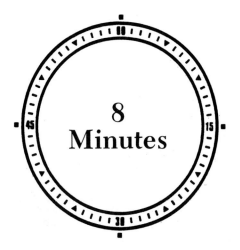

1 SHOULDER ARCH

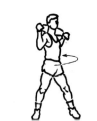

3 WAIST TWISTS

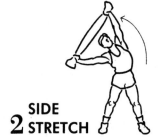

2 SIDE STRETCH

4 SHOULDER PULL

Someday Is Now

Your hard work and commitment have brought you to the point where exercise is part of your everyday life. That's why there is no formal graduation from *A Handle on Health*. Each time you exercise, it is like making a patch for the pattern of your life.

It might be tempting to put off making exercise a priority when you have achieved this much. But now that your body is currently operating as an efficient machine, it's a better idea to stay well-tuned. If you do "fall off the wagon," you can get back on by following this schedule.

If you don't exercise for more than three weeks, return to *The Maintain Program*. If the layoff is for more than six weeks, exercise in *The Train Program* for six weeks and progress to *The Maintain Program* for six weeks. If you stop your regular exercise routine for more than six months, begin with *The Gain Program* for the six-month progression.

On the other hand, if you feel you want more of an exercise challenge, try *The Competitive Edge* for six to eight weeks. You can switch back and forth between these two routines as your goals dictate and/or your schedule allows. Every day, you and those you live and work with will benefit from your handle on health.

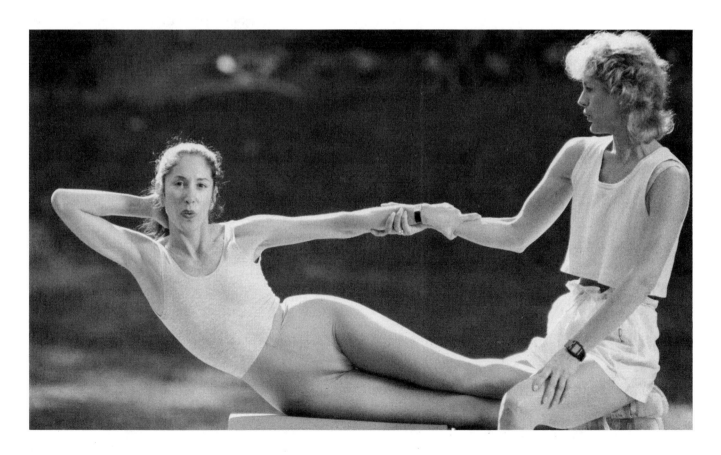

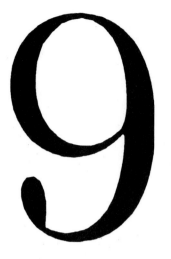

When you start this program, you have been exercising two or three times a week for six months, and have upper-range scores on the fitness assessments.

THE COMPETITIVE EDGE

You've earned the fitness you currently have. At this level looking good and feeling great is not an end in itself, but a means to perform better or sharpen your intellect. *The Competitive Edge* is where mind and body meet, where physical ability unleashes personal potential in a significant way. Agility, speed, balance, coordination, reaction time, and physical power are skills for success required in sport and in life. The executives I train are working on the same skills as the athletes. Only the arena of challenge is different.

If you look at exercise as an intermediate objective to a greater goal, this is the training program that will help you develop specialized skills. There are unique methods to emphasize your conditioning in both the aerobics and strength segments. If you are following this program, you undoubtedly possess the determination to set and reach your goals. This program gives you what you need to achieve *The Competitive Edge*.

Training Tips For The Competitive Edge

Strive for moderation. Keep to a steady routine for long-term gains instead of short-term performances.

Explore current fitness options. Consider stair running, rock climbing, backpacking, kayaking, bicycle touring.

Participate in leisure physical activity too. Try badminton, horseshoes, and nature walks.

Don't eliminate any segment of the workout. Always include flexibility, strength, and aerobic exercise in your one-hour workouts.

Remember to check your pulse. It's important to ensure you train at the prescribed heart rate intensity to produce results.

Allow the relaxation that improves concentration and mental performance to fill your life. While you are making physical changes, don't turn exercise into a high-pressure, tension-laden chore. Read a book, go to the movies.

Interchange aerobic modes frequently. Going from the bike to the rower, from the treadmill to swimming, will increase your aerobic capacity.

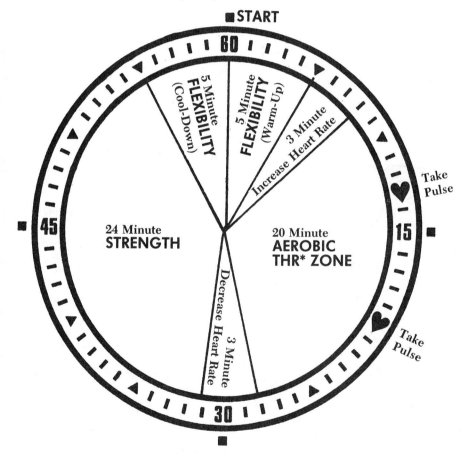

The Competitive Edge Exercise Hour

1 Hour Workout 3 times per Week and
45 min. of Aerobic Exercise 2 Days a Week

*Training Heart Rate

Warm-Up Stretches

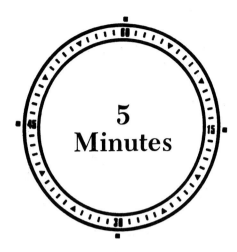

5 Minutes

Equipment

A mat or folded quilt and old bath towel.

Secrets of Stretching

● Warm up your muscles before stretching.
● Exhale as you stretch and inhale as you move into the next position.
● Stretch until you feel tension, then hold the position for 10 to 30 seconds.
● Avoid bouncing.
● Be precise when moving into position.
● Move smoothly and leisurely and *breathe*.
● Perform the stretches in the order listed.

Lower Body

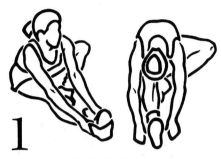

1

SINGLE LEG PULL (for back of leg) Bend forward from the hips, placing either your hands or a towel around the arch of the extended foot. Keep your back as straight as possible and bend the elbows as you exhale to increase the stretch. Put aside the towel and exhale as you lower the chest to the thigh. Throughout the stretch your foot points to the ceiling and hands slide alongside the extended leg.
● **Transition:** Raise your torso and bend the extended leg so you sit cross-legged.

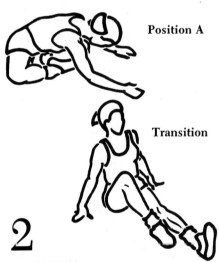

Position A

Transition

2

WIGWAM (for buttocks and lower back) Turn toward the inside leg and lower your upper body to the thigh. Arms are outstretched on either side of the knee.
● **Transition:** Roll up until you are sitting erect and facing forward. Place your hands behind you for support bringing the outside foot flat on the floor. Extend the inside leg with toes flexed to point toward the ceiling.

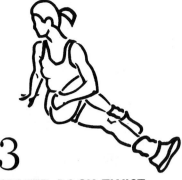

3

SEATED BACK TWIST (for entire back) Place the foot of the leg you have been working on the outside of the knee of the extended leg. Twist your torso toward the bent leg, placing your elbow on the outside of the bent knee. Balance your body with the fingertips of the hand behind you, exhaling as you pull that shoulder into a straight line with the forward shoulder. Be sure the hip of the side you are working is placed on the mat.
● **Transition:** Face forward and bring the soles of both feet together.

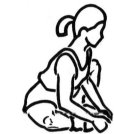

4

DOUBLE LEG PULL (for inner thigh) Taking hold of the toes of the feet, bring the elbows inside of the knees. Exhale as you bend the elbows pulling the upper body, with a flat back, toward the feet.
● **Transition:** Release your feet and roll slowly down to the floor and onto your back. Place the foot of the bent-knee leg on the floor and rest the foot of the stretching leg on the knee.

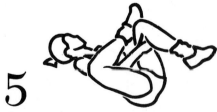

5

HIP STRETCH (for buttocks) Place your hands beneath the knee of the leg on the floor and exhale as you bend the elbows to pull the leg toward the shoulder. Keep the other leg relaxed and at a 90-degree angle to the knee.
● **Transition:** Stretch both legs flat on the mat and roll onto your stomach.

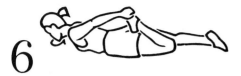

6

THIGH PULL (for top of thigh) Lying on your stomach, take hold of the foot with the hand on the same side of the body and pull the lower leg and foot to the buttocks.

● Transition: Release your grasp on the foot and place both hands under the shoulders with forearms flat on the floor, and head looking down at the mat.

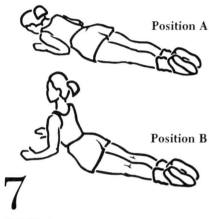

Position A

Position B

7

COBRA (for back and abdominals) Pressing the palms of the hands into the floor lift the upper body, without collapsing the shoulders, using the bent forearms to raise the torso while pelvis remains on the floor.

● Transition: Lower your torso until you are flat on the mat. Push yourself up until you are sitting on knees and feet.

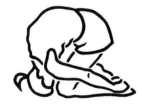

8

RABBIT (for upper back and top of shoulders) Place the crown of your head, the baby's "soft spot," onto the floor, as close to your knees as possible. Firmly wrap the palms of your hands around the soles of your arches. Deeply inhale, then exhale as you slowly lift the buttocks into the air while the arms straighten. You will feel this stretch in the upper shoulders.

● Transition: Roll upright until your torso is erect and hands are next to the knees.

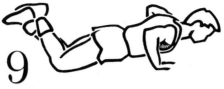

9

MODIFIED PUSH-UP (for chest) Resting on your hands and knees, position hands shoulder-width apart with fingers pointing forward. Keep your knees below the hip joints, your stomach muscles contracted and your feet lifted and crossed at the ankles. Lower your chest slowly as you inhale, touch the floor, then exhale as you lift to the starting position. Do sixteen repetitions.

● Transition: Push yourself up until you are sitting on your knees and feet.

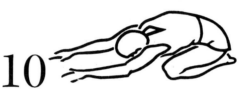

10

SLEEPING CAT (for lower back) Exhale as you bend from the waist and extend your arms out in front of you until your chest is on your thighs.

● First Transition: Roll over into a sitting position and start series with *Single Leg Pull* on the other side.

● Second Transition: Roll upright until your torso is erect and hands are next to knees.

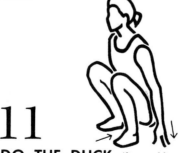

11

DO THE DUCK (for ankles and calves) With hands on either side, shift your weight until feet are shoulder-width apart and flat on the ground. Maintain the position while you stretch the lower leg.

● Transition: Shift weight to your knees.

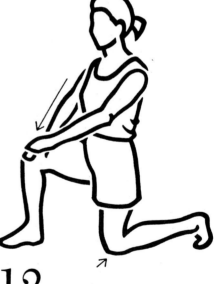

12

VERTICAL RISE (to protect back upon standing) Bring one foot forward so that your thigh parallels the floor. Place both hands on top of the knee in front of you, and pull the toes of your rear foot forward. Press down on the knee, stabilizing your balance as you stand up.

Aerobic Conditioning

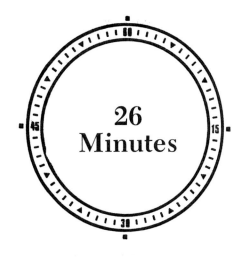

26 Minutes

Aerobic Training Tips

● Monitor your exercise intensity twice during each aerobic workout: Take your pulse at 8 minutes and 15 minutes into the activity.
● Take the time to learn the proper form and method for each activity.
● Move continuously for at least 20 minutes.
● If you exercise outdoors, accommodate to the weather.

Activity Swim, walk, cycle, rowing machine, dance exercise, cross-country ski-machine, jog, run, or a combination of these.

Intensity **3 minutes** to elevate heart rate—**20 minutes** in your personal heart rate zone—**3 minutes** to decrease heart rate to 100–110 beats per minute

Speed Work

Up until now the only type of aerobic training I have presented has been the continuous type. This has involved an aerobic warm-up of 3 minutes followed by a period of continuous activity in your training heart rate zone and perceived exertion range, ending with a 3-minute cool-down.

When intervals of exercise are interspersed with periods of recovery, it is called "interval training." This allows you to gain the benefits of higher intensity activity, which is increased aerobic power and speed. In fact, interval training is often called "speed work."

You begin an interval training session with your aerobic warm-up of 3 minutes. Increase your pace to the upper end of your training heart rate zone or your perceived exertion of 12–16. Hold that pace for 30 seconds to 5 minutes, depending on the workout. Then recover with low-intensity aerobic activity for a period of time at least equal to the interval duration at high intensity. You may have as little as three 5-minute intervals in one session to as many as ten 30-second intervals. The session will then end with a 3-minute cool down in which your heart rate should return to 100–110 beats per minute.

Interval Training Sequence

1. **Warm-up:** 3 minutes
2. **Maintain steady state:** after 7 minutes check training heart rate
3. **Start Intervals**
   Slow down: (slow pace or 1 mph) below training heart rate speed, for 1–2 minutes
   Increase speed: (increase pace or .5–1 mph) above normal training heart rate speed for 30–60 seconds
   Decrease speed: (slow pace or 1 mph) below normal

training heart rate speed for 30–60 seconds

4. **Repeat Intervals:** in sets of 4 repetitions with 1–2 minutes at your slow speed between the sets, and check heart rate

5. **Cool-Down:** 3–5 minutes to 110 beats per minute

The Competitive Edge Heart Rate Chart

	beats per minute—10-second count	
Round Up to Nearest Age and Resting Heart Rate		(RPE Scale) 12–16
Age	Resting Heart Rate	Competitive Edge 70–90%
20 years	60	158–186 **26–31**
	70	161–187 **27–31**
	80	164–188 **27–31**
30 years	60	151–177 **25–30**
	70	154–178 **26–30**
	80	157–179 **26–30**
40 years	60	144–168 **24–28**
	70	147–169 **25–28**
	80	150–170 **25–28**
50 years	60	137–159 **23–27**
	70	140–160 **23–27**
	80	143–161 **24–27**
60+ years work less than 80%	60	130–140 **22–23**
	70	133–142 **22–24**
	80	136–144 **23–24**

Interval Training Pointers

● Check your heart rate to make sure you are in your training zone. If you are over your heart rate, decrease the interval speed; if you are under your heart rate, increase the interval speed.

● Increase interval speeds as your fitness level improves by taking your heart rate and perceived exertion. Note the speed at which you are working to achieve your training heart rate and perceived exertion.

● A lower resting heart rate is the true test of improvement in fitness. As your fitness level improves, increase speed and decrease the amount of slow time during intervals.

Strength Training

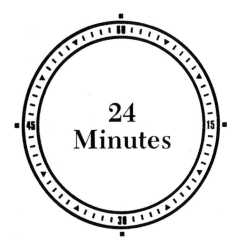

24
Minutes

Equipment

- 8, 10, or 12, and 15-pound dumbbells for women
- 5-pound ankle weights
- 10, 12, or 15, and 25-pound dumbbells for men
- A jump rope
- Flat exercise bench
- "Record your Workout" chart

Strength Training Secrets

- Pay attention to the execution of each exercise.
- Concentrate on the muscles you are using.
- Exhale on the contraction—the lift or push—and inhale during the opposite movement.
- Use slow, fully controlled movements in both directions without permitting momentum to do any of the work.
- Move through the complete range of motion that you can achieve.
- Keep exercises in the indicated sequence.
- Work up to 15 repetitions, then increase the weight of dumbbells by 2–3 pounds every 4 weeks.

The Competitive Edge

CHEST
1. **Chest Presses:**
   women 12–15-pound dumbbells, 8 reps × 1 set
   men 15–25-pound dumbbells, 8 reps × 1 set
2. **Flyes:**
   women 8–12-pound dumbbells, 8 reps × 1 set
   men 12–15-pound dumbbells, 8 reps × 1 set
3. **30–60 seconds of jump rope**

BACK
1. **One-Arm Rows:**
   women 10–15-pound dumbbells, 16 reps × 1 set
   men 15–25-pound dumbbells, 16 reps × 1 set
2. **30–60 seconds of jump rope**

SHOULDERS
1. **Pouring the Water** and
2. **Straight Arm Raises:**
   women 8–10-pound dumbbells, 8 reps × 1 set
   men 10–15-pound dumbbells, 8 reps × 1 set
3. **Lying Shoulder Lifts:**
   women 8–10-pound dumbbells, 8 reps × 1 set
   men 10–12-pound dumbbells, 8 reps × 1 set
4. **30–60 seconds of jump rope**
or
1. **Military Presses** and
2. **Upright Rows:**
   women 10–12-pound dumbbells, 12 reps × 1 set
   men 10–15-pound dumbbells, 12 reps × 1 set
3. **30–60 seconds of jump rope**

ARMS
1. **Alternate Curls** (each arm) and
2. **Concentration Curls** (each arm):
   women 10–15-pound dumbbells, 12 reps × 1 set
   men 15–20-pound dumbbells, 12 reps × 1 set
3. **French Curls** (each arm) and
4. **Kickbacks:**
   women 8–10-pound dumbbells, 12 reps × 1 set
   men 12–15-pound dumbbells, 12 reps × 1 set
5. **30–60 seconds of jump rope**

ABDOMINALS

Do one full set of each and then repeat sequence.
1. **Crunches,** 48 reps × 2 sets
2. **Curl-Ups,** 48 reps × 2 sets
3. **Bicycles,** 48 reps × 2 sets
4. **Pops,** 24 reps × 2 sets
5. **30–60 seconds of jump rope**

LEGS

Do one leg and then the other.
1. **Outer Thigh Lifts,** ankle weight, 64 reps × 1 set (each leg)
2. **Corkscrews,** ankle weight, 64 reps × 1 set (each leg)
3. **Inner Thigh Lifts,** ankle weight, 64 reps × 1 set (each leg)
4. **Sissy Squats,** 32 reps × 1 set

or

1. **Knee-ups,** ankle weight, 64 reps × 1 set (each leg)
2. **Stationary Lunges,** 8–15 lb. dumbbells, 12 reps × 2 sets (each leg)
3. **Calf Raises,** 48 reps × 2 sets

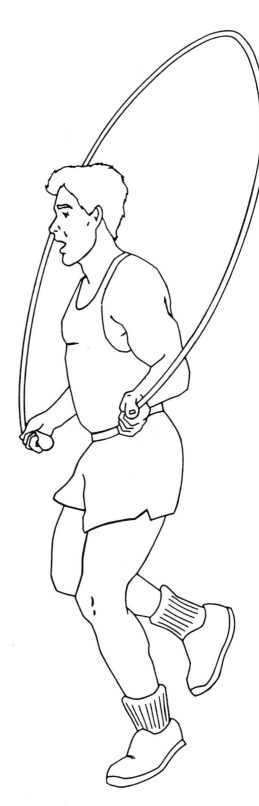

 For Aerobic Weight Circuit Training:
Between each major muscle group (i.e., between chest, back, shoulders, arms, and abdominals,) do 30–60 seconds of jump rope.

CHEST PRESSES Lie on your back on an exercise bench (a narrow sturdy coffee table or two ottomans pushed together will work) with feet on the bench, knees bent to keep your back flat, and dumbbells in both hands. Raise the dumbbells straight from the shoulder until arms are extended but elbows remain slightly bent. Inhale as you slowly lower the dumbbells to chest level, always keeping the forearms straight up at a 90-degree angle to the bench. Exhale as you push the bells overhead.

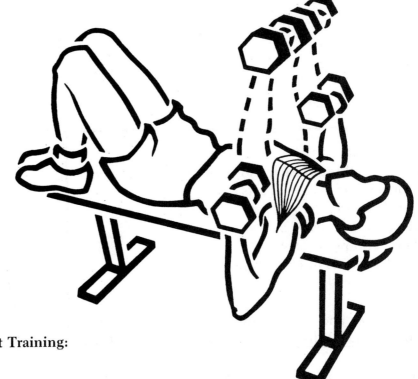

•

▶ For Aerobic Weight Circuit Training:
30–60 seconds of jump rope

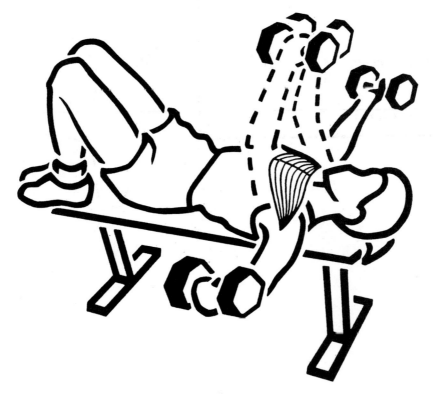

CHEST

FLYES Lie on an exercise bench with knees bent and feet on the bench to keep your back flat. Hold dumbbells over your chest with hands together, keeping your elbows slightly bent. As you inhale, lower the bells in a circular arc until they are level with your chest. Your elbows should be pointing to the floor but not lower than your wrists. Exhale as you raise the dumbbells to bring them together over your chest.

Position A

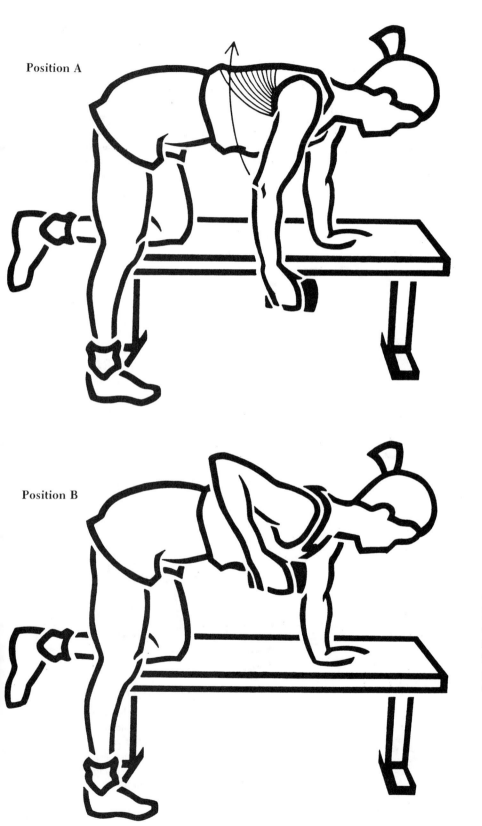

Position B

ONE-ARM ROWS Rest the arm and leg of one side on a low bench holding a dumbbell in the free hand. Keeping your shoulder immobile and your back flat, raise the weight straight up along the side of your body to just below the armpit. Exhale as you lift the bell, inhale as you lower it.

BACK

Position A   Position B

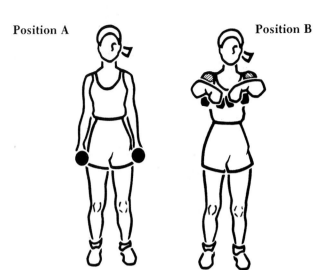

POURING THE WATER Stand tall with shoulders relaxed, hands at your side holding dumbbells, knees relaxed and feet about shoulder-width apart. Exhale as you raise your hands to chest level, palms down, and turn your hands slightly as if you're pouring water out of the ends of the bells. Keep elbows relaxed and bent. Straighten the wrists, then lower the bells to your sides as you inhale. Don't swing your arms—control those movements.

▶ You have a choice of exercises. Refer to your strength program chart.

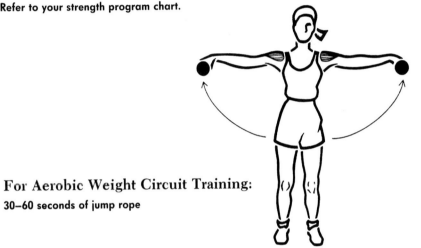

▶ For Aerobic Weight Circuit Training: 30–60 seconds of jump rope

STRAIGHT ARM RAISES With knees relaxed and feet shoulder-width apart, hold weights at your sides. Exhale as you raise dumbbells in an arc until arms extend straight out from the shoulders with wrists slightly bent. Return hands to your sides as you inhale.

Position A   Position B

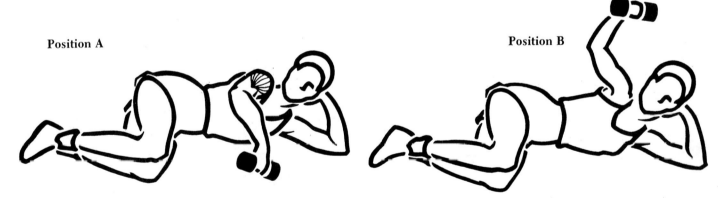

SHOULDERS

LYING SHOULDER LIFTS Lie on your side with knees bent, one hand supporting your head. Hold a dumbbell in the other hand in front of you, level with your shoulder. Exhale while lifting your arm straight overhead, keeping elbows and wrists relaxed. Inhale as you lower the weight.

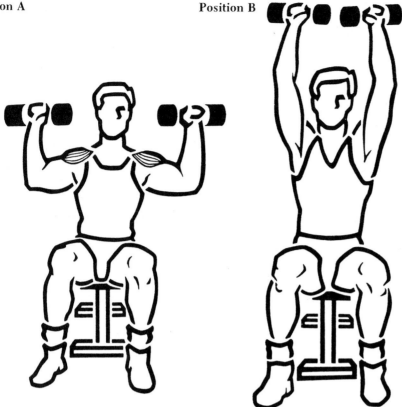

MILITARY PRESSES Hold dumb-bells above your shoulders, level with the ears. Arms will be L-shaped with shoulders relaxed. Slowly raise the bells straight up until arms are fully extended, but elbows are not locked. Do not arch your back or elevate your shoulders. Exhale as you lift and inhale as you lower the weights.

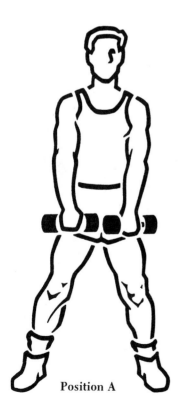

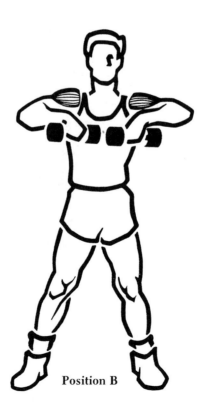

Position A   Position B

UPRIGHT ROWS Stand with your feet slightly farther than shoulder-width apart, knees slightly bent. Hold weights in front of thighs and lean forward slightly to avoid arching your back when you lift. With shoulders relaxed, bend your elbows to lift the dumbbells straight up to your collarbone. Exhale as you lift and inhale as you lower the bells.

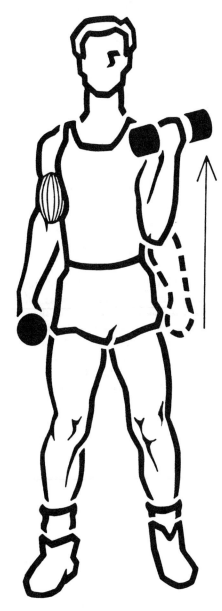

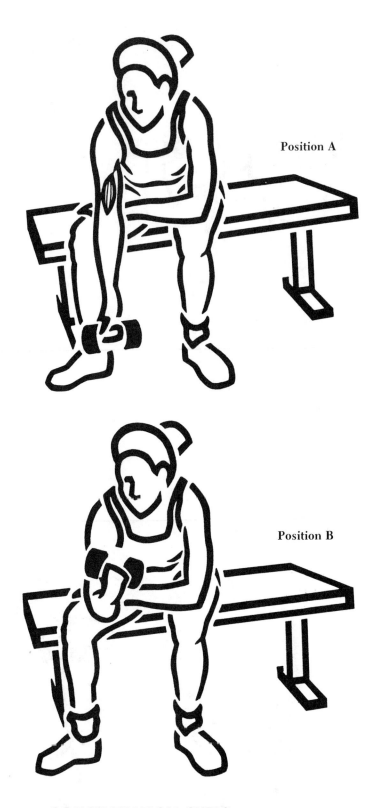

Position A

Position B

ALTERNATE CURLS Stand with your feet slightly farther than shoulder-width apart and knees slightly bent. Hold weights at your sides and lean forward slightly to avoid arching your back when you lift. Keeping shoulders down and elbows at your side, raise the forearm only to lift the weight to the shoulder. Lift one dumbbell at a time, alternating sides.

ARMS

CONCENTRATION CURLS Sit on a bench or chair. Leaning forward from the hips with a straight back, place one hand on the opposite knee. With the other hand, grasp a dumbbell and let your arm hang straight and relaxed. As you exhale, raise the weight by bending your elbow. Be sure that the shoulder doesn't drop and that the effort is felt in the arm, not the shoulder. Inhale as you lower the weight.

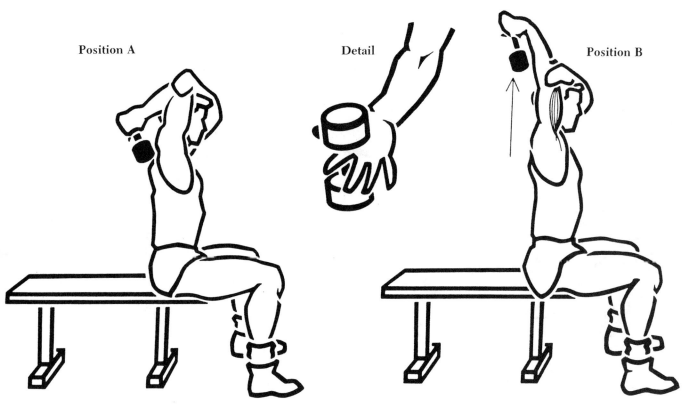

Position A
Detail
Position B

FRENCH CURLS Sit with feet apart and back straight, but not arched. Hold the end of the dumbbell in one hand (see detail) and use the other hand to steady the weight-bearing arm so the elbow remains pointing straight up near the ear. Raise your forearm overhead without locking the elbow, exhaling on the lift and inhaling as the dumbbell lowers behind your head. Be careful that the weight-bearing arm does not shift back and forth.

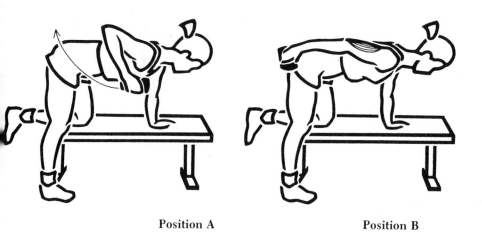

Position A
Position B

KICKBACKS Rest your knee and hand on a chair or bench. Keeping the back straight, grasp a light weight in the opposite hand and bring your elbow to waist level so the upper arm is at your side and the forearm hangs straight down. Keeping the upper arm immobile, exhale as you extend the lower arm in a straight line behind you. Bend your elbow to bring the weight to your shoulder and then extend it behind you again. Be sure that your wrist stays straight in line with the lower arm.

▶ **For Aerobic Weight Circuit Training:**
30–60 seconds of jump rope

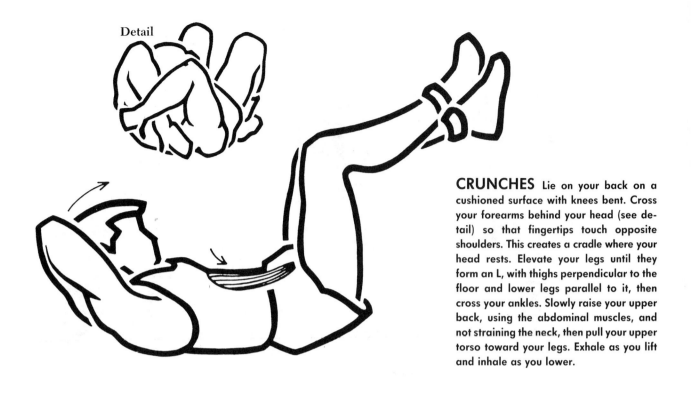

Detail

CRUNCHES Lie on your back on a cushioned surface with knees bent. Cross your forearms behind your head (see detail) so that fingertips touch opposite shoulders. This creates a cradle where your head rests. Elevate your legs until they form an L, with thighs perpendicular to the floor and lower legs parallel to it, then cross your ankles. Slowly raise your upper back, using the abdominal muscles, and not straining the neck, then pull your upper torso toward your legs. Exhale as you lift and inhale as you lower.

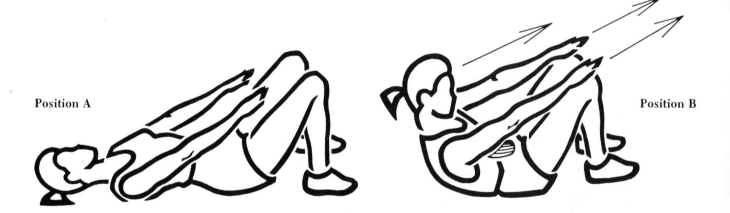

Position A

Position B

ABDOMINALS

▶ Do one full set of each and then repeat sequence.

CURL-UPS Lie on your back on a cushioned surface with lower legs at about a 90-degree angle with the floor and feet hip-width apart. Extend arms in front. Raise only your head and shoulders until the upper back is off the floor and your fingertips are on the thighs. Slide your fingers in a path along your thighs to the middle of your kneecaps, then lower your shoulders back to the floor. Exhale as you curl up and inhale as you return to the floor.

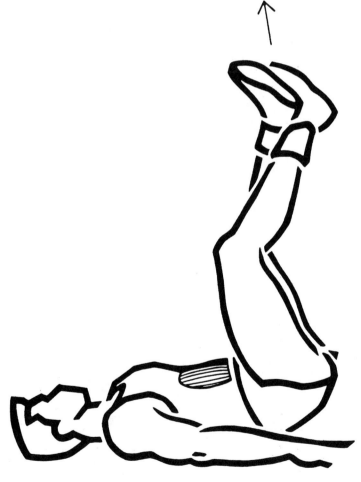

BICYCLES Lie on your back on a cushioned surface with hands behind head. Lift both legs into an L shape, keeping the lower leg parallel to the floor during the exercise. Raise your shoulders from the mat and alternately touch an elbow to the opposite knee while moving your thighs slightly back and forth. Keep your lower back pressed into the mat and contract your abdominal muscles to support the action. Touching the elbow to both sides is 1 repetition.

POPS Lie on your back, hands next to hips, palms down, legs straight up with knees slightly bent and ankles crossed. As you exhale, raise the buttocks one inch, then inhale as you lower the buttocks. Don't drop the hips sharply, but move slowly and steadily.

▶ **For Aerobic Weight Circuit Training:**
30–60 seconds of jump rope

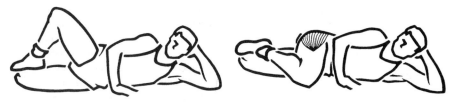

Position A   Position B

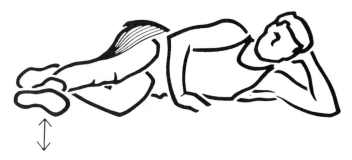

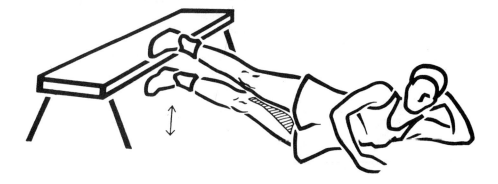

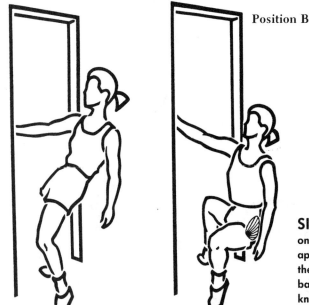

Position A   Position B

You have a choice of exercises.
Refer to your strength program chart.

OUTER THIGH LIFTS Lie on your side supporting the head with one hand while the other hand rests on the mat in front of your chest for balance. The leg against the floor should bend at the knee at a 45-degree angle, while the upper leg extends straight out from the body parallel with the thigh of the lower leg. Keeping your foot flexed so that the toes do *not* point, inhale as you lower the extended leg to the floor and exhale as you raise it to hip level.

CORKSCREWS Lie on your side with your head resting on one hand while the other supports your body by resting on the mat in front of your chest. Place the foot of your upper leg on the knee of the lower leg (as you get stronger, the foot will hang just above the knee). Slowly lower the knee of the upper leg toward the floor while you inhale, and return the knee as you exhale.

INNER THIGH LIFTS Lie on your side with one foot beneath a bench or chair and the upper foot resting on the chair or bench seat. Rest your head on one hand, place the other in front of your chest for balance. Exhale as you lift the lower leg to touch the bottom of the bench; inhale as you lower the leg to the floor. Raise and lower the leg with control.

SISSY SQUATS Stand at a doorway on the balls of your feet shoulder-width apart and toes pointed outward. Hold onto the door jamb at shoulder height and lean back the length of your arm. Bend your knees, lowering your buttocks halfway to the floor as you inhale. Push the pelvis toward the door, squeezing the buttocks, as you exhale.

LEGS

▶ Do one leg and then the other.

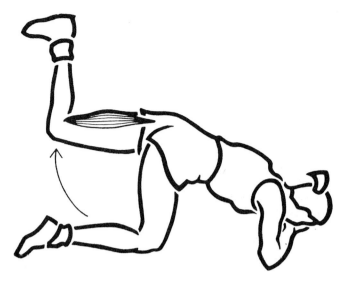

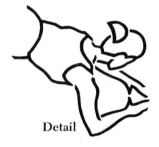

Detail

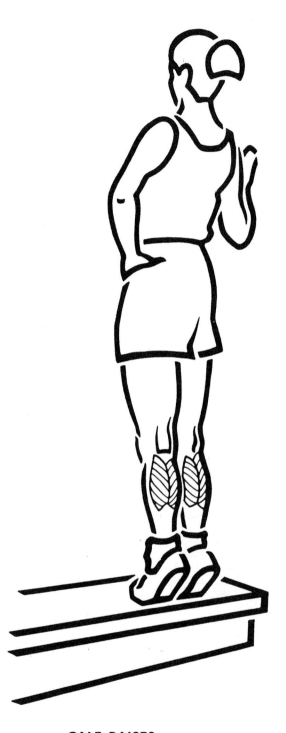

KNEE-UPS Rest on your elbows and knees with hands touching to form a triangle where your head can rest. Raise one leg until your thigh is parallel to the floor. The lower leg forms an *L*-shaped 90-degree angle. Keep your foot flexed so toes do not point. Lower this leg to the knee of the supporting leg as you inhale and raise it to hip level as you exhale.

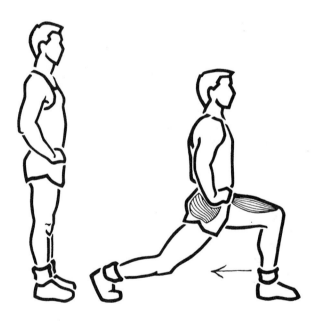

STATIONARY LUNGES Begin with feet together and hands on hips or holding dumbbells at your sides. If you need to practice, do them without weights until you have your balance. Keeping your torso erect throughout the exercise, take a giant step forward, transfer your weight to the forward leg, and sink until the thigh on the front leg is parallel to the ground while inhaling. The knee is directly over the ankle and the front foot flat on the floor. Exhale as you bring the forward leg back by pushing off the heel, until feet are together, returning to the starting position. Stay on the same leg for the entire number of repetitions, then switch to the other leg.

CALF RAISES Stand next to a wall using one hand for balance, with the balls of your feet together on a step or thick telephone book. Keeping knees straight but not locked, inhale as you slowly lower your heels toward the floor and exhale as you rise on the balls of your feet. Be sure that your ankles do not twist outward.

Cool-Down Stretches

5 Minutes

The Cool-Down stretches that end your workout are different than the stretches that began it. Follow them in the sequence shown.

Upper Body

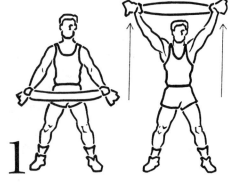

1

SHOULDER ARCH (for shoulders) Taking the towel in both hands, stand with your feet farther than shoulder-width apart with arms straight. Without locking your elbows, raise both your arms in an arc, keeping the towel taut, until hands swing behind the head. Lower your hands to the thighs and repeat the movement smoothly 5 times.

● Transition: Hold the last stretch above the head and bend the knees slightly.

2

SIDE STRETCH (for sides of the trunk) Keeping the towel taut, exhale as you use one hand to pull the towel downward, bending the trunk to one side. Prevent your back from arching by tightening the abdominal muscles. Increase the stretch for 3 deep breaths by pulling down on the towel with the lower arm, continuing to bend to the side. Slowly stand straight and repeat the stretch on the opposite side.

● Transition: Stand erect, knees slightly bent, towel over head. Bend your elbows, lowering the stretched-out towel behind your head.

3

WAIST TWISTS (for back and trunk) With toes and hips pointing straight ahead and abdominals tightened, anchor your hips by pressing the abdominal muscles toward the back. Twist your trunk slowly in one direction as far as you can without letting the hips turn. Hold the towel in a straight line to keep your elbows back, and face forward. Twist to the opposite side, then alternate sides 8 times.

● Transition: Face forward and release your grip from one end of the towel.

4

SHOULDER PULL (for shoulder) Extend the hand holding the towel straight in front of you. Your free hand, palm up, travels under the extended arm and hooks around the upper arm just above the elbow. Use the hooked arm to pull the straight arm toward the middle of your body. Hold for 3 breaths, then transfer the towel to the other hand and repeat the stretch on that side.

● Transition: Bring the hand holding the towel over your head, then bend your elbow so the towel is hanging to the floor behind you.

5

ARM PULL (for back of arm) Bring your free arm behind your back to grab the towel at a comfortable distance. The arm holding the towel should be near the ear with the elbow pointing forward. Pull down on the towel to stretch the back of the bent arm as you exhale. Hold the stretch for 3 deep breaths, keeping the tension in the towel constant. Then switch the towel to the other hand and repeat the stretch.

● Transition: Let go of the towel with the upper arm and extend both arms downward with palms facing toward the rear. Grasp both ends and stretch the towel behind your back.

6

CHEST PULL (for chest) Holding the towel in a straight line, lift both arms straight up until you feel the stretch in the chest and shoulder muscles. Take 3 deep breaths in this position while the muscles relax.

Lower Body

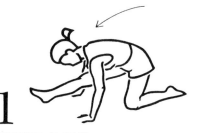

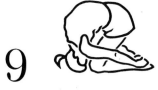

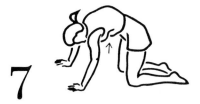

7

CAT AND CAMEL (for lower, middle, and upper back) Rest on hands and knees, making sure that the knees are under the hips and the hands are directly under the shoulders. As you exhale, round your spine, curling the torso away from the mat, and press your stomach toward the back. Inhale as you lift your head and gently lower the pelvis. Don't overarch your back. Exhale as you round the spine again. Alternate these 3 times.
● Transition: Return to starting position.

9

RABBIT (for upper back and top of shoulders) Place the crown of your head, the baby's "soft spot," onto the floor, as close to your knees as possible. Deeply inhale, then exhale as you slowly lift the buttocks into the air while the arms straighten. You will feel this stretch in the upper shoulders.
● Transition: Roll upright until your torso is erect and hands are next to the knees.

11

FORWARD BOW (for back of leg) Bending from the waist, exhale as you lower your chest toward your thigh. Be sure you are not sitting back, but that your stabilizing knee is directly under the hip, and your buttocks are over the knee.
● First Transition: Pull back the forward leg to bring both knees together. Start series with the *Modified Lunge* on the other side.
● Second Transition: After completing the series on the opposite side through the *Forward Bow* pull back the forward leg to bring both knees under you.

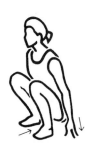

12

DO THE DUCK (for ankles and calves) With hands on either side, shift your weight until feet are shoulder-width apart and flat on the ground. Maintain the position while you stretch the lower leg.
● Transition: Shift weight to your knees.

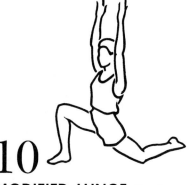

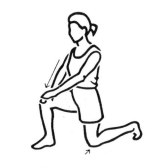

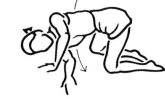

8

BACK BRIDGE (for middle back) Roll one shoulder onto the mat while both knees remain on the floor. Keep the knees under your hips and extend one arm, palm up, under the bridge formed by your body. Push into the shoulder with the arm that is stabilizing the bridge so that you feel the stretch between the shoulder blade and the spine. Exhale as you intensify the stretch, then repeat on the other side.
● Transition: Straighten your shoulders, then sit on your heels. Firmly wrap the palms of your hands around the soles of your arches.

10

MODIFIED LUNGE (for front of leg) Using the muscles in your thighs, move one foot forward until the knee is perpendicular to the floor and in line with the heel. Move the pelvis forward to stretch the back leg. The back thigh should form a 45-degree angle with the floor, and the top of the foot should be flat against the mat. Adjust your front foot to keep the knee over the toe. Raise your hands over your head, keeping the torso erect as you exhale. If you need to stabilize your balance place both hands on the front knee.
● Transition: Inhale as your pelvis moves backward to straighten your forward leg, and place your hands either on your knee or on the mat for balance.

13

VERTICAL RISE (to protect back upon standing) Bring one foot forward so that your thigh parallels the floor. Place both hands on top of the knee in front of you, and pull the toes of your rear foot forward. Press down on the knee, stabilizing your balance as you stand up.

Best Is More

I'm reversing the outdated exercise saying that "more is better." A body of scientific research has proven that is not true for exercise. But what *is* true is this: Best is more. When you perform exercise with precision, participate in a variety of activities, exercise consistently and at the appropriate intensity, then you will be rewarded by the utmost that exercise can provide.

The Competitive Edge is the perfect program to follow when you're training for sports, a half-marathon race, or are seeking marked physique changes. You can use it at any time to achieve a specific goal, which can take six to eight weeks. Then switch to *A Handle on Health* for your maintenance fitness plan. By alternating between the two, you can be innovative in designing a program that will keep you fit through the years.

A planned and purposeful exercise program is the method for achieving a powerful body—and a healthy body. That's what will help you keep your competitive edge.

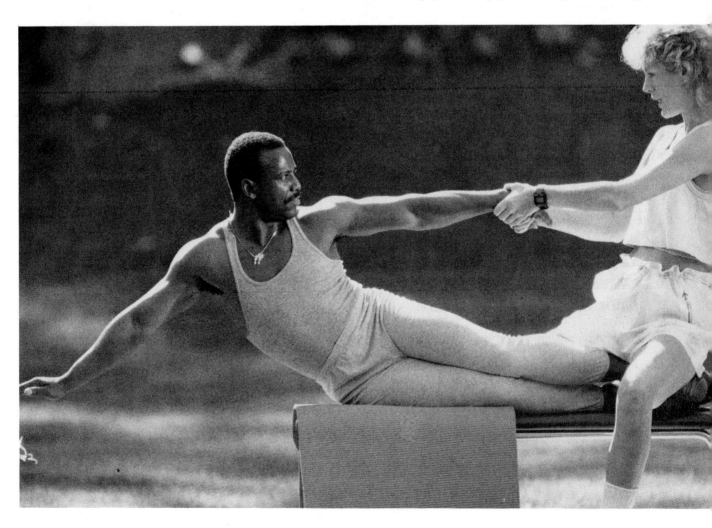

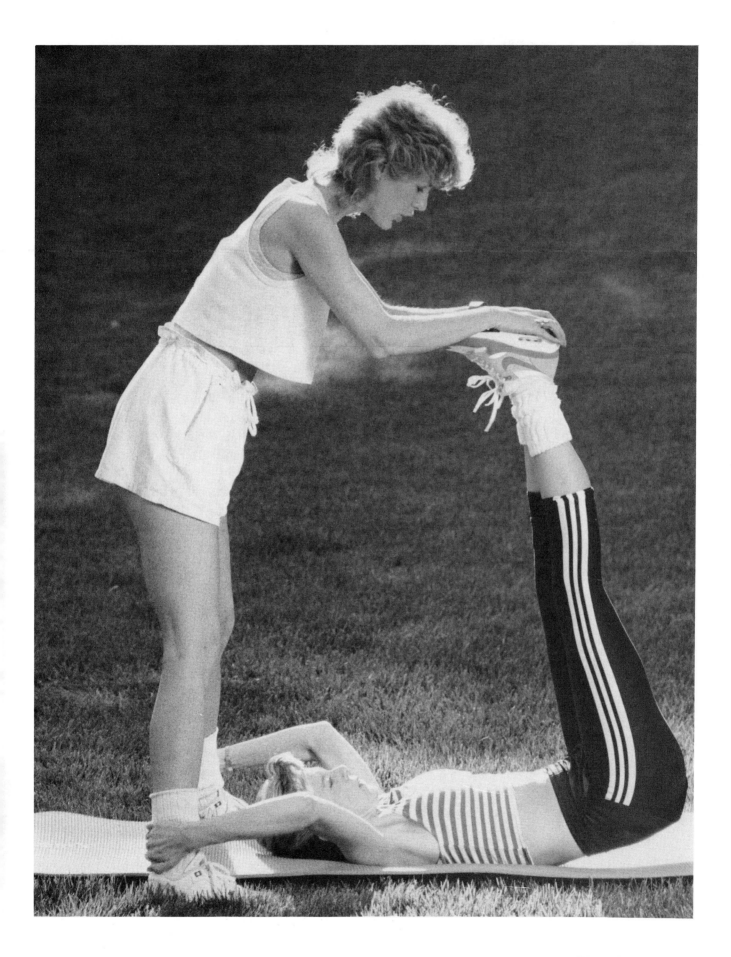

10
THERE'S FITNESS IN YOUR FUTURE

"Where do you see yourself one year from today?"

That's the question I ask each of my clients during our first meeting. Most reply that they want to lose so many pounds, or gain so much in muscle. That's fine as far as it goes.

"Do you want to be exercising on your own?" I prompt.

Most clients tell me that once they've learned how to exercise effectively they can foresee a time when a regular fitness routine will become a natural part of their life-style. Perhaps the strongest motivation to exercise on your own will be the time and money it will save you. Retaining a personal trainer for any length of time can be costly. Depending on the frequency of your sessions with a personal trainer, prices can range from $7,000 to $22,000 a year. A realistic and attainable goal for you, and all of my clients, is to achieve a maintenance-conditioning level from the Full Circle Fitness program within one year. My goal is to help you rely on yourself, so that after you have progressed to this level, exercise will become a regular part of your weekly routine as well as a lifetime commitment.

If you want to get the most value from a personalized fitness program, you must absorb the fundamentals of how to exercise. Blindly following directions and remaining oblivious to exercise know-how will not put you in charge of your personal program. However, if you apply the principles presented in the first four chapters of this book, you can execute a productive fitness program and become your own personal trainer.

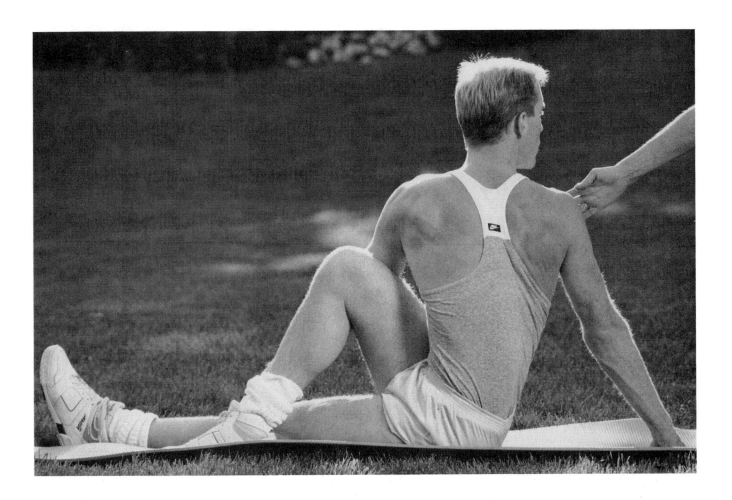

The way people react to this kind of independence is a lesson in human nature. Some people tend to avoid taking action. Lacking physical confidence, they will simply go through the motions without remembering to practice correct form or sequence, nor will they monitor their heart rate. These people usually put off self-motivated exercise and life-style changes of all kinds.

Others try to take on too much exercise in too short a period of time and believe that they know it all. They want to charge through each session, even at the very beginning. Chargers totally change their diets overnight and often buy a surplus of exercise equipment before structuring a realistic program. These people tend to exercise too hard too frequently, and don't bother to monitor their intensity. By progressing too soon, they can end up with needless pain, frustrations, or injuries.

But after several weeks or months of following Full Circle Fitness programs, both groups of people generally learn how to exercise effectively and perform sound exercise technique. It may take one person longer than another,

Fitness Tips For Your Future

- If you fall off the fitness wagon hop back on! Recognize that you will probably miss an exercise hour or splurge on ice cream every now and then, because your body is seeking its former status quo. Don't torture yourself when this happens, just jump back into your program.
- Include friends and family as "training partners." Plan time for exercise so that it fits into the whole family's schedule. This will go a long way both to cut down resentment over "lost" hours and to make physical fitness activities a family affair. Invite new health-minded friends, who support your current goals and make activity fun, into your social network.
- Change happens between you and yourself. Your performance at work will undoubtedly improve as exercise and weight-loss enhance your mental clarity and boost your energy. Not all of your co-workers will appreciate this change, and perhaps some will try to sabotage your efforts with nonsupportive remarks or actions. This kind of backlash generally wears itself out. In the meantime, stick with your program and simply ignore negative comments.
- Seize an opportunity for spur-of-the-moment activity. You can make the most of your lunch hour by spending half of it on a walk one or two days a week. When you're driving, or waiting at a red light, try pressing your abdominals into your back. If you're in the habit of joining co-workers for appetizers and drinks after work, counteract the "gut rut" by inviting work pals to make exercise class or nine holes of golf the "happy hour."

but eventually everyone learns their own exercise program as well as how to vary their routine; consistent exercise trains brains as well as muscles. In the meantime, eating moderate but filling amounts of nonfat foods and replacing potato chips with apples becomes less of a chore the more it's done.

Changes in attitude and habits sound simple when you read about them, but even the smallest change can be difficult. The body and mind are set in their ways, as the cliché goes, and it takes an active effort to move beyond the comfort of old habits. No matter how good your intentions are, or how clear-cut the foreseeable rewards, your body, family, and friends may resist your newfound healthful lifestyle in both subtle and obvious ways.

Use Your Mental Muscle!

How do successful exercisers achieve their fitness goals? Determining those goals is an important first step. They must be specific and should be attainable in the short and the long run. It works best to put a time limit on your goals, such as losing one pound a week or twenty pounds in three months. Choosing your direction is the first step in getting there.

One of my clients plans on paper; she makes grocery lists, to-do lists, and lists of all the gear she needs for trips. She finds that keeping a three-ring binder on her desk with a monthly workout schedule, workout records, fitness-assessment charts, and a training diary make her commitment to regular exercise easier. In one column she sets her goals, then she records her exercise routine. She also allots extra space in her records for any miscellaneous comments or reminders she might care to note. Writing everything down works for her as well as if she had an actual training partner.

Visualization is a tool that is frequently used by athletes and successful businesspeople such as Alice. When she arrives for a session, Alice visualizes how she will look and feel after she has completed her warm-up stretches. Before the aerobic phase, she visualizes the end of the twenty-minute session, and while she's doing her strength exercises, she envisions the completion of her reps. Visualizing helps Alice maintain her concentration as well as savor the sense of accomplishment that comes at the completion of the hour.

Your mind does not distinguish between a negative and a positive thought—it believes what it hears. If you start an exercise thinking "Oh, no, this is horrible, I'll never finish these reps," or "I'm too tired," then you may be setting yourself up for failure even if you have more than enough physical capacity to accomplish the exercises. Also, you won't have any fun. That's why Alice visualizes the positive end result of the exercise hour.

Positive thinking is a hackneyed term, but it *can* work. When Harold joined the program he was very overweight and sedentary, and he started denigrating his looks the moment I saw him. Since exercise requires effort, he would launch into jokes about "fat guys" as an excuse for not even trying. To help change Harold's self-fulfilling prophecy, I assessed his fitness capacity and took his measurements every six weeks. Proof of his progress helped Harold realize that he had the power to change for the better. Plus, during a session, Harold was encouraged to really *feel* the exercise and push away the negative thoughts. To make a long story short, Harold has shed those undesirable pounds and is successfully maintaining his desired weight range. He has dramatically changed his self-image and now records his workouts and monitors his progress with a regular fitness assessment.

Food For Health

My clients often want to know what kind of diet they should go on. That's not surprising since many people start exercising to control their weight. But it is difficult to determine, from the vast number of fad diet books currently on the market, which program is the best to follow. My response is, "Don't diet, think of food as fuel, and eat for energy!"

I counsel my clients to select a wide variety of foods from the four basic food groups to ensure that they consume the essential nutrients to support an active life-style. The word *diet* encompasses *all* the foods we eat. An eating plan is designed to help you manage the amount of food you eat so that you can control your weight and remain healthy. In order to both maintain an optimal weight range and enjoy your food, you can adjust your dietary intake to the energy you expend.

For anyone who desires good health and successful weight control, realistic eating and regular exercise go hand in hand. I suggest that my clients follow eating principles developed by reputable dietitians and medical doctors. The Low-Fat—High Energy eating plan is not faddishly popular, but it works, and that is what counts in the long run.

Low-Fat High Energy

It is recommended that of the total number of calories you ingest, you take in the following percentages of carbohydrates, fats, and proteins.

● 55–58% Carbohydrates
(48% should be complex carbohydrates and foods that contain natural sugars, such as vegetables, grains, cereals, bread, beans, and fruit. Only 10% of the carbohydrates you eat should contain refined and processed sugar.)

● 12–15% Protein
(Fish, fowl, meat, eggs, beans, tofu, yogurt, nuts, seeds, low-fat dairy, and certain combinations such as rice and beans)

● 30% Fat
(Whole milk, most cheeses, butter, margarine, nuts, meats, and polyunsaturated cooking oils)

Diets that provide less than 1,000 calories per day are not successful on a long-term basis. When you take in fewer than 1,000 calories per day, your metabolism acts as if you are entering a state of semi-starvation. Continuing to follow such a restricted diet will result in a marginal nutritional intake, an emotional state of deprivation, a weight-loss plateau, boredom, and a reinforced sense of failure.

Food Tips for Healthy Eating and Dietary Control

Be sure to eat a breakfast high in complex carbohydrates (cereal, bread, fruit, whole grains). If you don't, you'll get ravenous later on and overeat. Also, your body needs fuel to function at its best, and your brain needs complex carbohydrates to stay sharp.

Eat fruit instead of downing a quick glass of juice. If you want fruit juice and need to reduce your intake of calories, dilute your juice with water, seltzer, or low-sodium sparkling water.

At lunch, eat substantially and make it the main meal of your day. For example, eat a broiled chicken breast with steamed vegetables and a small salad with lemon juice. You can give yourself variety the next day by having pasta, a mixed green salad with rice vinegar or low-calorie dressing, and a slice of whole-grain bread for lunch.

If you don't recognize it, don't eat it! Eat all foods in their most natural form. For example, eat a raw apple instead of apple sauce, and a baked potato instead of mashed potatoes with gravy.

Eat color. The more intense the color of the fruit or vegetable, the higher its vitamin and mineral content will be. Do not eat anything white unless it is fish, chicken, or low-fat dairy. Avoid white flour, white rice, white bread, etc.

Reach for a mid-afternoon snack and pull out the apple or orange you keep at work or at home. Avoid so-called health-food snacks such as nuts, raisins, and dried fruits. They are high in fat, salt, or sugar. Choose a fast walk around the block instead of a walk to a sugar-filled vending machine.

Eat lighter at night. Think small. Big is not better for you or your guests' health. Emphasize vegetable dishes, salads, and non–milk-based soups. Remember, a potato is a low-fat, highly nutritious friend, but gobs of butter and sour cream turn it into a high-fat, high-calorie saboteur.

When you eat out, don't order from the entrée menu. These are usually large portions so they are high in calories. Instead, order side dishes a la carte, such as a plain baked potato and a vegetable plate.

Drink plenty of water throughout the day. Be sure to have water in convenient locations, such as in your car, on your desk, in your workout area, next to your bed, and by your side when you travel by airplane. Drink 6 to 7 glasses of water a day to keep a good fluid balance in your body.

Eat fresh foods for the vitamins you need. These vitamins help to translate foods into fuel. If you are concerned about your nutritional intake, consult a reputable dietitian or have a blood analysis done before taking vitamin supplements. The appropriate combination of essential nutrients is provided by a diet that contains food from a variety of sources. Plus, a balanced diet will give you the energy you need to keep exercising.

Eat fiber because it stimulates the intestinal muscles and helps regulate the absorption of the nutrients you ingest. Whole-grain breads, cereals, fruits, vegetables, and legumes provide you with a natural source of fiber. Additional bran can be taken with other foods, but it should always be taken in moderation.

Acknowledge a food craving. I allow my clients one "cheat" per week. If it's high in fat, salt, or sugar, and if it contains, or has been processed by, chemicals, it qualifies as "emotional" food. It's better to have the food you had as a child to quell frustration, fear, or anger than to suppress it with an entire package of bran muffins. The next day, get back to steamed, broiled, and fresh foods.

Enroll in cooking classes to enhance your repertoire of spices, herbs, and healthful dishes. This will add interest and variety to your daily cuisine. To make a healthy eating plan a reality you can also find plenty of delicious recipes in cookbooks.

For those of you who want to reduce your weight, the most successful means of achieving and maintaining your dietary goals is with this equation: One pound of fat is equal to 3,500 calories. Therefore, a daily deficit of 500 calories will result in a weight loss of one pound per week. A daily dietary reduction of 250 calories, combined with aerobic exercise that expends 250 calories per day, will result in a 3,500-calorie reduction over seven days. Faster weight loss is generally due to loss of water or lean body tissue such as muscle, not body fat.

Of course, I know it is easier to talk about than to follow a path of moderation when eating, but by being *aware* of what you are eating and by exercising consistently, you will achieve a steady weight loss. Plus, you will eat enough calories from a variety of foods to get the mix of nutrients you need to keep those extra pounds off permanently.

Remember that healthful food is not necessarily boring food, and that all meals, no matter how modest or health-oriented, are meant to be enjoyed and shared with family and friends.

Lose Fat Not Muscle

A simple method is used to determine the number of calories needed to maintain or achieve a specific weight. Multiply the weight you desire by the number under your sex and activity level.
EXAMPLE: Moderately active male, desired weight 165 lbs. = 165 × 16 = 2,640 calories per day

	Inactive	Moderately Active	Highly Active
Women	10	12	14
Men	14	16	18

(reprinted by permission of The American College of Sports Medicine)

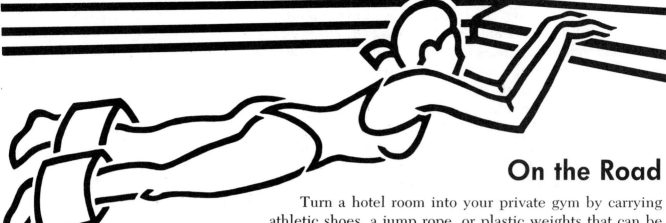

Water Exercise

On the Road

Turn a hotel room into your private gym by carrying athletic shoes, a jump rope, or plastic weights that can be filled with water from the bathroom tap in your suitcase. Stretches, crunches, push-ups, and lunge walks need no equipment. If you prefer, walk briskly around the town you are visiting or run up and down the hotel stairs for your twenty-minute aerobic conditioning. An increasing number of hotels are adding gyms, or establishing cooperative arrangements with nearby health clubs, to serve hotel guests. Maintaining your exercise program is the best way to guarantee energy for sightseeing or tough business negotiations.

Seek out vacations that feature adventure and activity. Rafting down rivers, hiking through mountains, cutting trails for the Sierra Club, or challenging your prowess in an Outward Bound program are a few alternatives that supply plenty of action. The most obvious aspect of trips like these is that you are out moving and doing rather than sitting around and eating out of boredom. Perhaps less obvious is the personal strength that comes from pushing yourself a little beyond what you think you can do. I recommend planning a weekend activity for each season, to get to "the great outdoors" and see all the natural wonders that are accessible to you.

Once you have a six-week base of consistent whole-body exercise, you can try a split-training routine. Do the 20- to 31-minute aerobic phase of the exercise hour first thing in the morning before taking a shower, then stretch for 5 minutes, and start your business day. On a split-training day, you can do your 20- to 24-minute strength-training routine at lunch with dumbbells at the office, or at least you can do a circuit of push-ups, crunches, and lunge walks. If this isn't feasible, then do the strength routine at night and do your 10- to 15-minute stretch routine before bedtime. This split-training exercise hour is an alternative routine for people whose "too busy to exercise" excuses threaten to derail their long-range goals.

Spa Spins

Throughout the year I offer special week and weekend trips, called Spa Spins, to Aspen and Europe (France, Switzerland, and Italy) or to resorts like Palm Springs and Santa Catalina Island, to get away from it all. A small group of clients and I hike through fields of wildflowers to breathtaking mountain slopes, where we can watch birds maneuver against clear skies as we do our stretches, crunches, and push-ups on meadow grasses. Beginning with a hearty breakfast of oatmeal and fruit, we spend the days hiking, swimming, stretching, and sharing ideas about fitness life styles.

The hikes can be quite challenging for people who are used to walking on level ground, but the purpose of Spa Spin is to remove us from what we're used to. By inviting extra effort and accomplishing it, we can leap enormous physical and mental barriers as well. Imagine savoring the exhilaration of walking ten miles instead of feeling exhausted just by thinking about it! When you do more than you think you can, it gives you the confidence and the energy to take on new challenges. Remember the principle of overload? When you work at higher levels than you normally encounter, your muscle strength and endurance capacity will improve. It works for the mind as well as the body.

A Final Word

The Full Circle Fitness program you select is determined by your *present* activity level; this is the *safest* way to start exercising on your own, to increase your capacity for exercise, and to maintain a program of regular exercise. Whether you are turning twenty-one or seventy-one, whether you are overfat or underweight, if you get tired just walking the dog, or if you can effortlessly complete a twenty-mile walkathon, there is a Full Circle Fitness program for you. Your desire to make a change is the essential ingredient of your success.

Throughout my years as a personal trainer, I have seen more than two thousand clients experience the surge of energy, stamina, relaxation, and health that comes from regular exercise and appropriate eating. May you too enjoy Full Circle Fitness as one of the many activities that makes a happy and full life, and may you endow your loved ones with a legacy of wellness and vitality.

Day Hiking

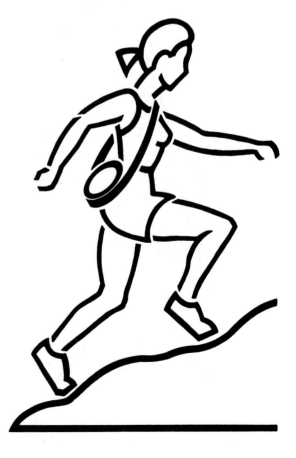

Appendix

FITNESS TESTS, CHARTS, AND RESOURCES

We can measure your physical fitness with the timed walk or step test, flexibility, and muscle endurance tests. These tests are not strenuous, but if you become uncomfortable, short of breath, extremely fatigued, or dizzy during any of them, stop and consult your doctor.

The timed walk and step tests are accompanied by a table to compare yourself to others of your sex and age. Maintain your perspective though, by not emphasizing your comparison to others, but rather by comparing your own personal progress over time.

The Timed Walk Test

In the *Timed Rockport Fitness Walking Test*, you will walk for one mile and then compare your time and pulse rate to the charts on pages 142–144. The results of this test depend on your pacing ability and degree of body fat.

To take the *Rockport Fitness Walking Test:*

1. Record your heart rate: If you do not know how to take your heart rate, use the following simple procedure and practice a few times.

Walk in place for 30 seconds, then place your index and second finger together on your wrist, your throat, your temple, or directly over your heart. If you use your wrist, place your fingers gently over the radial artery just inside the wrist bone. If you have trouble finding your pulse there, try inserting your fingers softly into the side of your neck at the level of the Adam's apple just below your jaw. Don't press too hard, because this can slow your heart rate and give you an inaccurate reading.

Count your pulse for 15 seconds and multiply by 4 to determine the beats per minute.

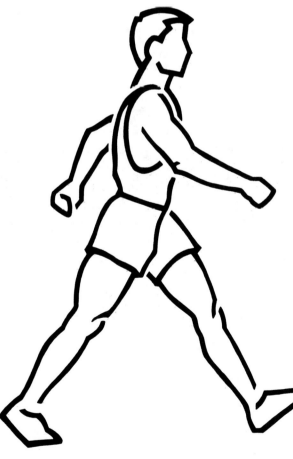

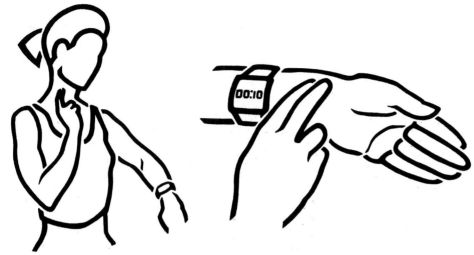

2. *Find a measured track or measure out a mile on your own.* Most high schools have ¼-mile tracks around their football fields, while recreational facilities have indoor tracks ¹⁄₁₆ of a mile or longer. You can measure out a mile along a flat road (without stop lights) by checking it against your car's odometer. Make sure that the path is an accurately measured mile.

For safety's sake, don't take the walking test outdoors when the temperature is above 85 degrees Fahrenheit or below 20 degrees, or when the air is heavily polluted. You may have to walk early in the morning to avoid heat and humidity.

3. *Walk one mile as fast as you can.* Before you start, take 5 minutes to stretch your muscles and be sure to wear proper exercise footwear and loose fitting clothes.

4. *Record your time.* Walking speeds vary greatly. Most people walk between 3.5 and 5.5 miles per hour, which means that one mile usually takes somewhere between 9 and 17 minutes.

5. *Take your heart rate.* Begin counting with the next full beat starting with 0. Count the number of beats in 15 seconds and multiply by 4 to determine the beats per minute.

6. *Record your heart rate immediately at the end of the mile.* This will give you all the basic information you need to know to determine your level of fitness now.

7. *Turn to the appropriate Rockport Fitness Walking Test chart for your age and sex marked Relative Fitness Level.* This chart will tell you how your results compare with individuals of your age and sex. For example, if your coordinates place you in the "above average" section of the chart, you're in better shape than the average person in your category. These norms for fitness levels were established by the American Heart Association.

Before the Tests

- Wear loose, comfortable clothing and athletic shoes.
- Do not smoke, drink coffee, or eat for two hours.
- Do not consume alcohol for eight hours.
- Do not exercise before you take the fitness assessments.

You Will Need

- A watch with a second hand, a digital watch, or a stopwatch.
- A cloth tape measure.
- A bathroom scale.
- A sturdy box and a 12-inch ruler or yardstick.
- Record your results on page 151.

How To Use the Timed Walk Charts:

Mark the point on the chart defined by your walking time and heart rate at the end of the walk. After you have recorded your walking time and heart rate, go along the horizontal axis (for "time") until you reach the point that represents how long it took you to walk the mile. Draw a line **straight up** from this point. Then go up the vertical axis (Heart Rate beats/min.) until you find the point representing your rate. Draw a line **straight across** from this point. The section in which the two lines intersect on the chart represents your relative fitness level.

The charts are based on weights of 170 lbs. for men and 125 lbs. for women. If you weigh substantially more, your relative cardiovascular fitness level will be slightly overestimated. If you weigh substantially less, your relative cardiovascular fitness level will be slightly underestimated. Record your results on the Personal Fitness Progress Chart on page 151.

Key:

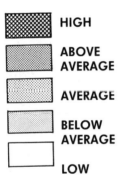

- **HIGH**
- **ABOVE AVERAGE**
- **AVERAGE**
- **BELOW AVERAGE**
- **LOW**

Relative Fitness Levels*

20-29 YEAR-OLDS

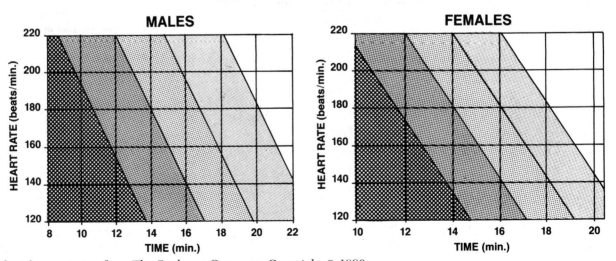

*reprinted with permission from The Rockport Company. Copyright © 1986.

30-39 YEAR-OLDS

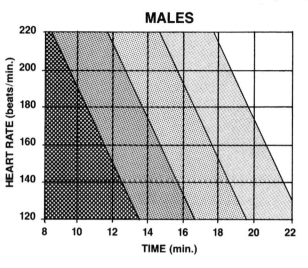

MALES

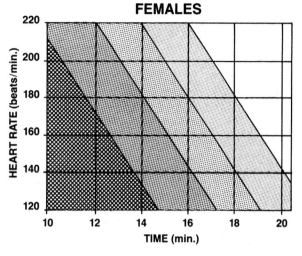

FEMALES

40-49 YEAR-OLDS

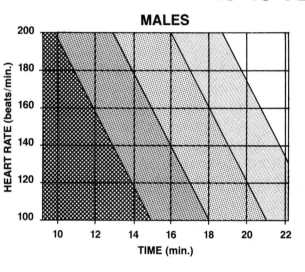

MALES

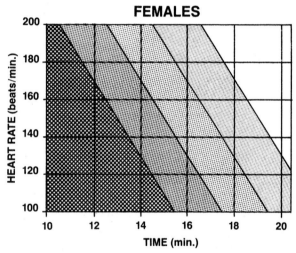

FEMALES

50-59 YEAR-OLDS

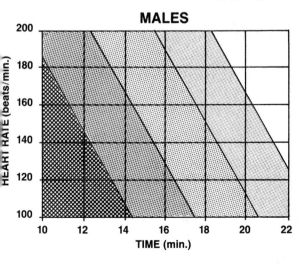

MALES

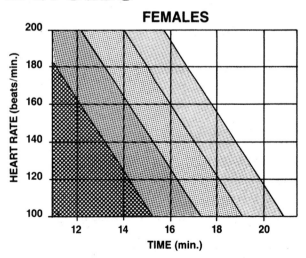

FEMALES

60 + YEAR-OLDS

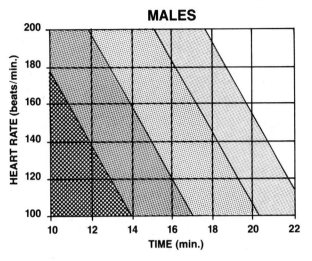

MALES

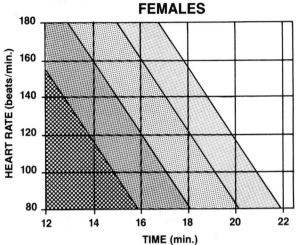

FEMALES

The Flexibility Test

This test will help you evaluate your range of motion when stretching your lower back and legs. If you have been sedentary, walk for 3 minutes before testing flexibility to warm up your muscles.

To take the Trunk Flexibility Test:

1. Sit with your legs fully extended and the bottom of your feet flat against a box projecting from the wall. The box should be the same height as your feet. With outstretched arms, hands on top of one another, bend slowly forward from your waist as far as possible. Hold the position at least 3 seconds. If you have had low-back discomfort or injury you may want to modify this test by bending the knees slightly or using a rolled towel under the knees. You may want to repeat this a few times and average your total.

2. Have a partner measure in inches the distance that you can reach before or beyond the edge of the box. Distances before the edge are listed as negative scores; those beyond the edge as positive scores.

3. Record your results on page 151 and compare your progress over time.

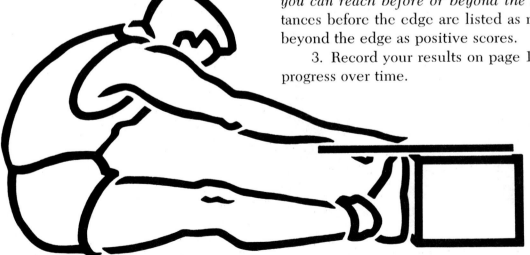

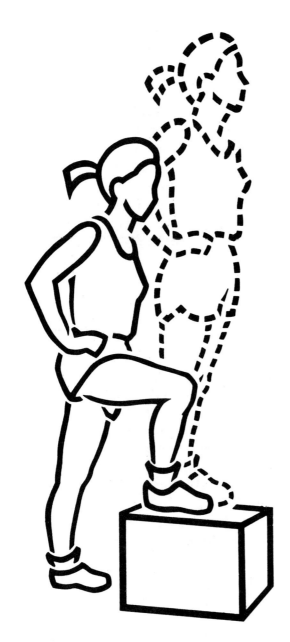

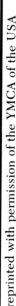

STEP TEST RATING SCALE		
35 Years and Younger		
1-minute Post-Exercise Heart Rate	Males	Females
Excellent	81	79
Good	99	94
Above average	103	109
Average	120	118
Below average	123	122
Fair	127	129
Poor	136	137
36–45 Years Old		
1-minute Post-Exercise Heart Rate	Males	Females
Excellent	84	79
Good	98	90
Above average	112	106
Average	120	118
Below average	125	125
Fair	129	134
Poor	138	145
46 Years and Older		
1-minute Post-Exercise Heart Rate	Males	Females
Excellent	90	87
Good	102	90
Above average	111	108
Average	120	118
Below average	124	124
Fair	130	130
Poor	138	145

The Timed Step Test

How to perform the test:

1. First step up with your right foot.
2. Then up with your left foot.
3. Down to the floor with your right foot.
4. Then down with your left foot (you may alternate with the lead foot if you desire).
5. Step for 3 minutes doing 24 cycles (up, up, down, down) per minute.
6. Stop and immediately count your pulse for 1 minute.
7. Compare your pulse rate according to sex and age in the table provided.
8. Record your results on page 151.

You Will Need

- A 12-inch step (the ideal step is a sturdy wooden box 12 inches high, 18 inches wide, and 10 inches deep, or a stack of firmly wrapped newspapers 12 inches high).
- A stopwatch or clock with a second hand.
- Some method of keeping a 96 beat-per-minute cadence. (A metronome is the ideal method of maintaining a stepping rhythm, or use your tape recorder by recording a "Go" and 3 minutes of the 96-beats-per-minute rhythm. End this recording with "Stop! Count your pulse for one minute.")

The Muscle Endurance Tests

Each of these tests lasts only one minute. You count the number of times you can do each exercise within those 60 seconds. If you haven't been exercising at all, it may be difficult to do even one. That's not at all unusual. But keep trying and do the best you can.

Although these are familiar exercises to most people, please read the instructions carefully. The correct form is critical for your safety, and these exercises have been updated since high school gym days.

Make sure you get clearance from a doctor before taking these tests if you have any history of heart disease or musculoskeletal problems. If you have pain while doing these tests, stop.

Curl-Up Test The purpose of this timed test is to evaluate abdominal strength and endurance. Lie on your back on a folded towel or blanket with arms at your sides, knees bent, feet flat on the floor, and heels about six inches from the buttocks. Raise only your head and shoulders. Extend your arms so that your fingertips are on the top of your thighs. When you raise your shoulders, exhale and try to touch the middle of the kneecap, and then return to the starting position. Do as many as you can in 60 seconds without pausing.

Timed Curl-Up Rating Scale
(number of repetitions in 60 seconds)

Men less than 50 years old
Low—less than 20
High—40+

Women less than 50 years old
Low—less than 16
High—36+

Men 50 and older
Low—less than 15
High—30+

Women 50 and older
Low—less than 11
High—26+

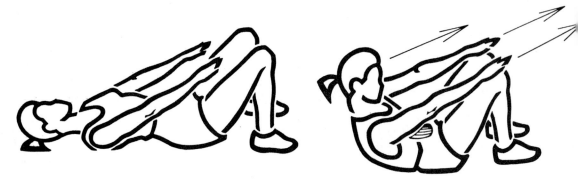

Position A   Position B

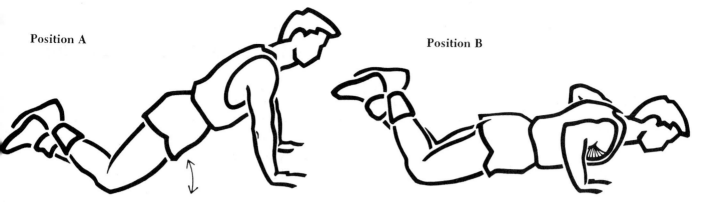

Position A

Position B

Modified Push-Up Test The purpose of this test is to evaluate upper body (chest, anterior shoulder, and arm) muscle strength and endurance. This modification of a standard push-up involves pushing up from the knees rather than the toes. Keep shoulders, back, and buttocks in a straight line, hands directly under shoulders, and knees bent. Bend elbows until your chest touches the floor, then exhale as you push up. Without pausing, do as many as you can within 60 seconds.

Timed Modified Push-Up Rating Scale
(number of repetitions in 60 seconds)

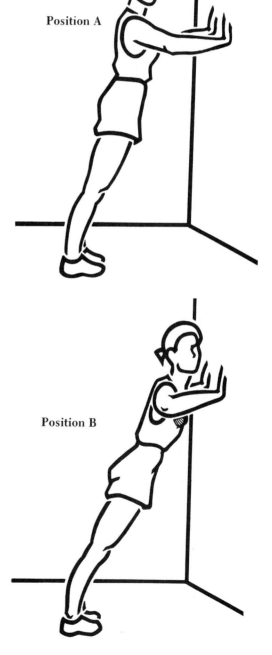

Position A

Position B

Men less than 50 years old	**Men 50 and older**
Low—less than 19	Low—less than 9
High—41 +	High—31 +
Women less than 50 years old	**Women 50 and older**
Low—less than 8	Low—less than 4
High—36 +	High—26 +

If you are unable to do one full push-up, use the wall push-away.

Wall Push-Away The purpose of this timed test is to compare your progress over time until you can perform the modified push-up test. Stand an arm's length away from a wall with hands at chest level (nipple line), palms flat on the wall, and fingertips toward the ceiling. Move your feet one or two steps farther away from the wall. With your head turned to one side and back held rigid, move your body in one unit, letting your elbows move to the side until your chest comes near the wall. Immediately, without resting, exhale and push away from the wall to the starting position. Do as many as you can within 60 seconds.

Record your results on the Personal Fitness Progress Chart on page 151 and compare your progress over time.

Record Your Workout

I've designed a workout chart for you (see next page) that includes these items: **Date—Aerobic—Chest—Back—Shoulders—Arms—Abs—Legs—Goals**

Use it to keep notes on every aerobic and strength workout and create your own workbook to make record keeping convenient. The record includes a column for your fitness goals so that you can make sure your program—and your progress—stay on course.

A quick way to keep these notes is with exercise shorthand. Once you learn this simple method, you'll be able to record your workouts quickly and easily.

Taking Notes for Aerobic Training: When recording your aerobic activity, note these four variables:

Activity (aerobic mode)
Duration (how long)
Distance (how far or # strokes)
Intensity (heart rate and perceived exertion)
—Record your training heart rate at 15 minutes like this: hr 25 = heart rate, 25 beats per 10 second count

Aerobic Shorthand = What Occurred

Bike/30'/5m hr 25/pe 12	=	*Bike*, 30 minutes, 5 miles, 10-second heart rate and perceived exertion
XC/15' hr 28/pe 14	=	*Cross-Country machine*, 15 minutes 10-second heart rate and perceived exertion
Run/30'/3 m hr 23/pe 11	=	*Run*, 30 minutes, 3 miles 10-second heart rate and perceived exertion
TM/20'/3.5 m. hr 19/pe 9	=	*Treadmill*, 20 minutes, 3.5 miles/hr 10-second heart rate and perceived exertion
Row/26'/600 hr 24/pe 10	=	*Rowing Machine*, 26 minutes, 600 strokes 10-second heart rate and perceived exertion
Walk/30'/2m. hr 18/pe 7	=	*Walk*, 30 minutes, 2 miles 10-second heart rate and perceived exertion
Swim/30'/800m hr 24/pe 12 OR	=	*Swim*, 30 minutes, 800 meters 10-second heart rate and perceived exertion OR
Swim/700m/7 × 100 hr 27/pe 14	=	*Swim*, 700 meters broken into 7 laps with a 30-second to one-minute rest 10-second heart rate and perceived exertion
LIA/20' w/w hr 22/pe 11	=	*Low-Impact Aerobics*, 20 minutes, wrist weights 10-second heart rate and perceived exertion

Taking Notes for Strength Training The shorthand sample below is a quick method for strength notetaking. When recording resistance, remember these three numbers in this order:

1. Amount of weight
2. Number of repetitions (how many)
3. Number of sets (a defined number of repetitions, i.e., 10 reps equal one set)

CHEST	p.u. push-ups c.p. chest press	10×2= (10 reps, 2 sets) 8/15×2= (8 lbs, 15 reps, 2 sets)
BACK	1 arm R 1 arm row	10/15×2= (10 lbs, 15 reps × 2 sets)
SHOULDERS	m.p. military press	12/10×2= (12 lbs, 10 reps × 2 sets)
ARMS	C Krl Concentration Curl	8/15×2= 8 lbs, 15 reps × 2 sets
ABS	CR (75) crunches	25×3= 25×3 sets = 75 crunches
LEGS	lng walk 10 corks corkscrews	10 lunge walks 2/25×2= 2 lbs, 25 reps, × 2 sets
GOALS	get started, 100 crunches, take fit tests end of week	

Sample Longhand Workout Record

Date	Aerobic	Chest	Back	Shoulders	Arms	Abs	Legs	Goals
1/1/90	Bike 20' hr. 25	incl p.u 8×2	1 arm R 5/8×2	water 3/8×2 raises 3/8×2	C Krl 5/8×2 k.b. 3/8×2	curl-ups 8×2 cr 8×2 1 leg 8×2	circles 8+8 outer 24 inner 24	GET STARTED
1/3	Walk 20' hr. 21	'' ''	'' ''	water 5/8×2 raises 5/8×2	C Krl 5/8×2 k.b. 5/8×2	'' ''	lng walks 16 calf rse. 16	keep at it

Blank Chart for a Training Notebook

Date	Aerobic	Chest	Back	Shoulders	Arms	Abs	Legs	Goals

Your Personal Fitness Progress Chart

	Today's Date	6 Weeks Date	12 Weeks Date	6 Mos Date	9 Mos Date	1 Year Date
Measurements						
Chest (at nipple line)						
Biceps (middle of upper arm at widest point)						
Waist (At narrowest point)						
Hips (4 inches below navel)						
Thighs (measure at halfway distance between kneecap and thigh socket)						
Knee (in sitting position, knee straight)						
Ankle (at narrowest point)						
Weight						

Fitness Assessment

Timed Walk Test						
Step Test						
Sit and Reach (inches)						
Curl-Ups (no./60 sec.)						
Modified Push-Ups (no./60 sec.)						
Wall Push away (no./60 sec.)						
Resting Heart Rate (beats per minute)						

Full Circle Fitness Resources

Audio Cassettes

Companion audio workout cassettes are available through Full Circle Fitness Products for four of the exercise programs in this book, plus a program to use for a workout on the road. All cassettes come with an illustrated manual and cost $11.50 per tape. A package of 5 cassettes costs $50 plus $2 shipping.

The Gain Program: This initial conditioning phase emphasizes all three components of exercise. The Gain Program tape is particularly good for those who have been inactive and want to get started on weight loss, increase flexibility, and improve muscle tone and stamina.

The Train Program: This is an improvement conditioning phase that progresses the occasional exerciser to an intermediate level. The Train Program tape is particularly good for the exerciser who wants to achieve moderate weight loss as well as increase stamina, strength, and flexibility.

The Maintain Program: A challenging workout for the regular exerciser, the Maintain Program tape intensifies the improvement phase of fitness training in order to achieve maintenance conditioning.

A Handle on Health: Maintenance conditioning begins six months after the start of regular exercise. Once this desired level of fitness is achieved, this tape will help maintain body weight, modify health risks, relieve stress, and encourage consistent exercise habits.

Fitness Tests and A Workout on the Road: A no-equipment routine that travels with you, it provides stretches and strength exercise, to do while you arc away from your fitness club or home gym.

The Computer Program

The PC Training Partner is a companion to the book that includes all five exercise programs on one disk. It has been designed to assist you in recording your workouts, and to progress you through beginning and improvement conditioning to a lifestyle of regular exercise. The PC Training Partner is IBM compatible and features a multi-user capacity. It costs $74.95 plus $3 UPS shipping.

The audio cassettes and computer program are available by mail. California residents add 6.5% sales tax. Make check or money order payable to Full Circle Fitness Products, 1018 West El Norte Parkway, Suite #142, Escondido, California 92026.